Ready Note

to accompany

The Psychology of Physical Activity

Albert V. Carron
University of Western Ontario
Heather A. Hausenblas
University of Florida
Paul A. Estabrooks
Kansas State University

Boston   Burr Ridge, IL   Dubuque, IA   Madison, WI   New York   San Francisco   St. Louis
Bangkok   Bogotá   Caracas   Kuala Lumpur   Lisbon   London   Madrid   Mexico City
Milan   Montreal   New Delhi   Santiago   Seoul   Singapore   Sydney   Taipei   Toronto

McGraw-Hill Higher Education

A Division of The McGraw-Hill Companies

Ready Notes to accompany
THE PSYCHOLOGY OF PHYSICAL ACTIVITY
ALBERT V. CARRON, HEATHER A. HAUSENBLAS, PAUL A. ESTABROOKS

Published by McGraw-Hill Higher Education, an imprint of The McGraw-Hill Companies, Inc., 1221 Avenue of the Americas, New York, NY 10020. Copyright © The McGraw-Hill Companies, Inc., 2003. All rights reserved.

This book is printed on acid-free paper.

2 3 4 5 6 7 8 9 0 QPD QPD 0 3

ISBN 0-07-284962-2

www.mhhe.com

Chapter 1: The Psychology of Physical Activity

The Psychology of Physical Activity
Albert V. Carron
Heather A. Hausenblas
Paul A. Estabrooks

The journey of a thousand miles starts in front of your feet
Lao-Tzu

A Tomato's Tale

The Tomato Effect

➡ a term used to describe a phenomenon whereby highly efficacious therapies are ignored or rejected.

➡ Why does it occur?
  ➢ Because the therapy does not seem to make sense in light of popular beliefs or common understandings.
  ➢ Because people simply ignore the evidence available

A Tomato's Tale

☼ From its origins in Peru the tomato played a significant role in the diet of most Europeans by 1520.

☼ However, in North America Tomatoes were considered poisonous.

☼ Because of the dominant popular belief, tomatoes did not enter the North American Diet until 1820

_____

_____

_____

_____

_____

_____

_____

Does Physical Activity suffer from a tomato effect?

1. Is physical activity an efficacious therapy?

2. Does society in general avoid physical activity?

3. Are people aware of the benefits of physical activity?

_____

_____

_____

_____

_____

1. Is Physical Activity an Efficacious Therapy?

☼ Chronic physical activity positively influences health ....

➡ The skeletal system
  ➢ Bone density in youth
  ➢ Likelihood that bone mineral density will be retained in older adults.

➡ The muscle system
  ➢ Hypertrophy
  ➢ Strength and endurance
  ➢ Capillarization & maximal blood flow.

_____

_____

_____

_____

_____

_____

1. Is Physical Activity an Efficacious Therapy?

➡ **The cardiovascular system**
- ➤ Cardiac mass
- ➤ Stroke volume and cardiac output
- ➤ Heart rate and blood pressure (lower)

➡ **The respiratory system**
- ➤ Ventillatory-diffusion efficiency while active

➡ **The metabolic system**
- ➤ Triglycerides (decreased)
- ➤ Adiposity (decreased)
- ➤ High density cholesterol
- ➤ Insulin-mediated glucose uptake

How much Physical Activity is necessary?

🔔 **Basic Requirements:**
- ➡ 30 minutes or more of moderate intensity performed on most days of the week.
  - ➤ Ventillatory-diffusion efficiency while active

🔔 **Benefits are related to effort:**
- ➡ Additional benefits are associated with increased intensity or duration of the activity.

---

2. Is Physical Activity Avoided?

🔔 **National surveys have been conducted**
- ➡ Australia: National Health Foundation (1985)
- ➡ United Kingdom: Sports Council of Great Britain (1990)
- ➡ United States: U.S. Dept of Health & Human Services (1991)
- ➡ Canada: Fitness Canada (1981)

🔔 **Estimated percent who are active varies depending on the definition**

2. Is Physical Activity Avoided?

🔔 Any participation in one or more of 90 sports in last 12 months
  ➜ 68%**
🔔 3 or more hrs/wk during 9 or more months of the year
  ➜ Approx 56%**
🔔 3 or more kcal/kg per day
  ➜ 15 to 20%*

* Canada Fitness Survey
** Center for Disease Control Behavior Risk Factor Survey

---

2. Is Physical Activity Avoided?
A Comparison Across Nations

1. In which of the following countries are the most number of people moderate to highly active?

2. In which of the following countries are most number of people minimally active?

Australia	No. 2 in Physical Activity!!
Canada	No. 3 in Physical Activity!!
Finland	No. 1 in Physical Activity!!
United States	No. 4 in Physical Activity

---

3. Are People Aware of the Benefits of Physical Activity?

🔔 Godin, Cox, and Shephard (1984) queried physically active and inactive individuals about their knowledge and beliefs about physical activity.

🔔 In most instances, inactive individuals held similar beliefs to active individuals about the benefits of physical activity.

4

3. Are People Aware of the Benefits of Physical Activity?

☼ Inactive people agree that physical activity can be used to…
- ➡ control body weight
- ➡ be more healthy
- ➡ relieve tension
- ➡ improve physical appearance
- ➡ feel better
- ➡ meet people

☼ Yet they don't participate.

Does Physical Activity Suffer from a Tomato Effect?

☼ YES!!
- ✓ an efficacious therapy
- ✓ Society in general avoids physical activity
- ✓ People are aware of the benefits of physical activity

☼ How can the effect be reduce or eliminated?

☼ Through science that focuses on the psychology of physical activity.

Psychology of Physical Activity

☼ Devoted to gaining an understanding of

- ➡ individual attitudes, cognitions, and behaviors in the context of physical activity

- ➡ the social factors that influence those attitudes, cognitions, and behaviors

Historical Developments

☼ **Why has the science of physical activity psychology been slow to develop?**

➤ Traditionally, sport more popular

➤ Physical activity as modality for disease prevention and maintenance of general health not fully known until recently

➤ Traditionally, biomedical model followed = treatment of disease as opposed to its prevention

Definitions of Important Terms

☼ **Physical Activity**

➤ Any body movement produced by skeletal muscle that results in a substantial increase over the resting energy expenditure

☼ **Exercise**

➤ Planned, structured and repetitive PA designed to improve or maintain fitness

☼ **Physical Fitness**

➤ Person's ability to perform physical activity

Definitions of Important Terms

☼ **Health**

➤ A human condition with physical, social, and psychological dimensions

☼ **Active living**

➤ A way of life in which physical activity is valued and integrated into daily life

Related Areas of Interest

- Health vs. Physical Activity vs. Rehabilitative Psychology
- The dependent variable should be used as a main classifying variable
  - Smoking cessation = Health
  - Recovery from a car accident = Rehabilitative
  - Improved exercise adherence = Physical activity

END

Chapter 2: The Measurement of Physical Activity

The Psychology of Physical Activity
Albert V. Carron
Heather A. Hausenblas
Paul A. Estabrooks

It is a capital mistake to theorize before one has data
Sherlock Holmse

Measurement is the Heart of Science

☼ **Enables researchers and health-care professionals to:**

➡ Specify which aspects of physical activity are important for a particular health outcome

➡ Monitor changes in physical activity over time

➡ Monitor the effectiveness of an intervention

➡ Determine the prevalence of people guidelines for physical activity

What Should be Measured?

☼ **Type:**
  ➡ The main physiological systems that are activated during the activity

☼ **Frequency**
  ➡ The number of times a person engages in an activity over a pre-determined period of time

☼ **Duration**
  ➡ The temporal length of the activity

☼ **Intensity**
  ➡ The degree of overload an activity imposes on physiological systems in comparison to resting states

---

Important Measurement Issues

☼ **What are you measuring?**
  ➡ Physical Activity versus Energy Expenditure versus METs

☼ **Validity**
  ➡ The ability of a test to accurately assess what it is developed to assess.

☼ **Reliability**
  ➡ The ability of a test to yield consistent and stable scores

---

Important Measurement Issues

☼ **Feasibility**
  ➡ The practicality of the measure for its intended population

☼ **Objectivity**
  ➡ the ability of different testers to provide similar test scores for a given individual

Subjective Techniques to Assess Physical Activity

- ☼ **Typically paper and pencil questionnaires.**
  - → Easy to administer
  - → Relatively inexpensive
  - → Can be used to assess a large sample of individuals quickly

---

Self Report Measures

- ☼ **Godin's Leisure Time Physical Activity questionnaire**
  - → Assesses a typical week's strenuous, moderate, and mild physical activity
  - → Calculation for METS
  - → Validity and reliability data available
- ☼ **Advantages:**
  - → Speed and ease of administration
  - → Typical week
- ☼ **Disadvantage:**
  - → Reliability is questionable for mild and moderate activity

---

Self Report Measures

- ☼ **7-Day Physical Activity Recall**
  - → Assesses a previous week's moderate, hard and very hard physical activity
  - → Calculation for METS
  - → Validity and Reliability are strong
- ☼ **Advantages:**
  - → Speed and ease of administration
  - → Calculation of total energy expenditure
  - → Occupational and leisure activities.
- ☼ **Disadvantage:**
  - → Previous week may not provide typical participation

Self Report Measures

☼ **Lifetime Total Physical Activity Questionnaire**
- ➜ Assesses lifetime involvement in occupational, household, and exercise/sport physical activity
- ➜ Interview based with cognitive cues and recall calendars

☼ **Advantages:**
- ➜ Provides history

☼ **Disadvantage:**
- ➜ No strong validity data

Self Report Measures

☼ **Ratings of Perceived Exertion**
- ➜ Assesses single session intensity.

☼ **Advantages:**
- ➜ Good Reliability
- ➜ Good Validity

☼ **Disadvantage:**
- ➜ No frequency data

Self Report Measures-For Children

☼ **Early physical activity measures for children were completed by parents or teachers**
- ➜ Typically were not valid or reliable
- ➜ 7-Day Recall--invalid and unreliable

☼ **Previous Day Physical Activity Recall**
- ➜ Good Reliability

Self Report Measures-For Older Adults

☼ **Physical Activity Scale for the Elderly**
  ➔ Assesses a variety of physical activities of daily living
  ➔ Specific cues for older adults

☼ **Advantages**
  ➔ Quick to complete
  ➔ Good validity and reliability

Diary Methods

☼ **Typically completed at the end of each day**

☼ **Can be modified to specific behaviors**

☼ **Advantages**
  ➔ No need for observation
  ➔ Detailed information can be obtained

☼ **Disadvantages**
  ➔ Expensive to reduce the data to analyzable form
  ➔ Heavy participant burden
  ➔ Questionable validity due to tedium

Self Report Measures-Overview

☼ **Many questionnaires are available to assess physical activity**

☼ **However there is no gold standard for measurement**

☼ **All self-report measures are associated with error**

☼ **They are relatively effective indicants of which people are more or less active**

Objective Measures of Physical Activity

☼ Technology has only recently become available to objectively assess the minutes spent at different intensities of physical activity.

☼ Activity monitors have the potential to provide substantial benefits over self-report--they avoid the biases and inaccuracies of recall.

Pedometers

☼ Pedometers are simple movement device counters that can estimate habitual physical activity over a relatively long period.

☼ Less obtrusive devices
   → Light weight
   → clip onto a belt or are worn around the ankle

Pedometers

☼ Limitations with the reliability and validity of mechanical and electronic pedometers.
   → Low validity
   → Some devices show high deviations from the actual step rate

Accelerometers

- Caltrac
  - assesses vertical movement of the trunk which is one characteristic of walking and running
- Has adequate reliability for both children and adults

- Limitations
  - Bicycling, weight lifting skating, and swimming cannot be assessed well with the device

Heart Rate Monitors

- Can provide minute-by-minute data for up to 16 hours.
- Good validity
- Limitations
  - Heart rate monitors cannot distinguish accurately between light and moderate intensity activities
  - Elevated heart rates can be produced by mental stress in the absence of physical activity
  - Heart rate monitors can be inconvenient to use
  - Various electronic devices interfere with the recording resulting in lost data

Doubly Labeled Water

- Doubly labeled water technique considered by some to be the gold standard
- Measures energy expenditure
- Assessment of doubly labeled water requires that the participant ingest known amounts of hydrogen and oxygen isotopes.
- Energy expenditure can be calculated based on the difference between rates of loss of hydrogen and oxygen.

Doubly Labeled Water

☼ It is valid for children, adult, and elderly populations.

☼ Limitations

- ➡ Each dose of oxygen currently costs several hundred dollars and the analysis of samples requires a mass spectrometer, which costs about $250,000 U.S.
- ➡ Impractical for use in large epidemiological studies or in educational programs.
- ➡ The measure does not provide data on the type, frequency, intensity, or duration of physical activity.

Direct Observation

☼ Advantages:

- ➡ It is accurate
- ➡ It involves little inference with the participant's routine
- ➡ Diverse dimensions related to physical activity can be quantified
- ➡ It can be used as a criterion method for validating other measures of physical activity

☼ Limitations:

- ➡ It is time-consuming
- ➡ Observation is expensive
- ➡ Observations may not reflect habitual physical activity

END

Chapter 3: Cognitive Functioning and Physical Activity

The Psychology of Physical Activity
Albert V. Carron
Heather A. Hausenblas
Paul A. Estabrooks

Mens sana incorpore sano
Homer

Interpreting Research:An Example

- 50 studies vary in:
  - Sample size tested
  - The nature of the sample tested
  - Operational definitions
- 35 studies show ↑ fitness = ↓reduced anxiety
- 10 show fitness is unrelated to anxiety
- 5 show that ↑ fitness = ↑ anxiety

- What conclusion can be made from these studies?

Interpreting Research: An Example

- ☼ **Narrative review:**
  - ➡ An overview or summary that draws on general impressions
  - ➡ A narrative review would conclude that the research is inconclusive

- ☼ Meta Analysis?

Meta-Analysis

- ☼ Statistical summary of the results from the various studies.

- ☼ Results from individual studies are converted to an <u>effect size</u> = standard score

- ☼ Standard scores can be added and then averaged to draw conclusions about the overall impact of a particular treatment.

- ☼ A meta analysis would would indicate what the effect is <u>in general</u>

Interpretation of Effect Sizes

Small	Medium	Large
.30	.50	.80

Does exercising make you smarter?

Meta-analysis of Physical Activity and Cognitive Functioning

N = 134 studies
1, 260 effect sizes

PA has small beneficial effect on cog function (ES = .25)

Etnier et al. (1997)

Moderator: Physical Activity Type

Moderator: Study Design

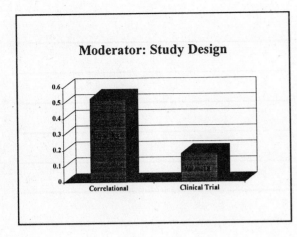

Moderator: Age

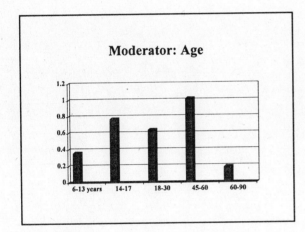

Moderator: Dose-Response

- No relationship between cognitive functioning and exercise:
  - → Session duration
  - → Frequency per week
  - → Program length

- Not able to provide prescriptions for doses of PA necessary to increase cognitive functioning

4

END

Chapter 4: Physical Activity and Mood

The Psychology of Physical Activity
Albert V. Carron
Heather A. Hausenblas
Paul A. Estabrooks

True enjoyment comes from activity of the mind and exercise of the body
Wilhelm von Humboldt

What is Mood?

※ A complex construct that is defined a number of different ways by different authors.

※ Negative Affect
➡ Anxiety, Depression, Fatigue, Anger, Confusion

※ Positive Affect
➡ Vigor, Pleasantness, Euphoria

Physical Activity and Anxiety

☼ **Anxiety**
- → A negative emotional state characterized by feelings of nervousness, worry, and apprehension
- → State versus trait

☼ **A number of meta analyses suggest a small to moderate effect of physical activity on anxiety reduction (ES=.15-.56)**

Anxiety and Physical Activity: Moderators

☼ **Task type**
- → Aerobic exercise=small effect
- → Anaerobic exercise=no effect

☼ **Dose-response**
- → Aerobic activity 0 to 20= ES .78
- → 20-40 minutes = ES . .31
- → > 40 minutes= ES . .28
- → Any intensity is related to reduced anxiety

☼ **Physical activity is as effective for anxiety reduction as other behavioral techniques used to manage the disturbance**

Physical Activity and Depression

☼ **Non-clinical Depression**
- → Listlessness, feelings of gloom

☼ **Clinical Depression**
- → Loss of interest, lowered mood, at least 2 weeks
- → At least 5 of the following:
- → Loss of appetite, weight gain or loss, sleep disturbance, decreased energy, psychomotor retardation , sense of worthlessness, guilt, concentration problems, thoughts of suicide

Physical Activity and Non-clinical Depression

※ Depression is reduced with physical activity

※ Effect of exercise varies from small to medium

Category of Subjects	Effect Size
High school students	.60
College students/faculty	.16

Exercise and Clinical Depression?

- Depression is reduced with physical activity
- Effect of exercise varies from medium to large

Source of Depression	Effect Size
Medical rehab	.97
Psychological rehab	.55

Depression and Physical Activity: Moderators

※ **Task type**
  ➔ Beneficial effects occur with all types of activities (weights, aerobics, walking, etc.)

※ **Dose-response**
  ➔ Longer the duration (wks.) the greater the benefit
  ➔ 9 weeks seems to be a threshold but effects are experienced immediately

※ **Combination of physical activity & psychotherapy provides best reduction**

Other Measures of Mood and Physical Activity

- Profile of Mood States (POMS)
- Negative moods:
  - anger, tension, fatigue, depression, & confusion

- Positive mood:
  - vigor

McNair et al. (1971)

POMS and Exercise

McDonald & Hodgdon (1991)

Why Does Exercise Benefit Cognitive Functioning & Psychological States?

- Cognitive explanations
- Physiological explanations

4

Cognitive Explanations

1. Expectancy hypothesis

Individuals expect to feel better so they report feeling better

Doesn't seem likely given physiology evidence

2. Distraction hypothesis

Exercise is time out from daily stresses

Time outs alone don't provide the same degree of benefit as exercise

Physiological Explanations

1. Thermagenic hypothesis

Increases in core temperature associated with reduced muscle tension

May account for anxiety reductions

Doesn't account for changes in cognitive functioning and/or depression

Physiological Explanations

2. Monoamine hypothesis

Exercise is a stimulus that increases level of neurotransmitters (I.e., dopamine, norepinephrine, serotionin)

Neurotransmitters facilitate neural impulses across synapses.

Could account for effects of exercise on anxiety, depression, cognitive functioning

Physiological Explanations

3. Opponent process hypothesis

    Human system works to stay in balance (homeostasis)

    A stimulus (pleasurable or aversive) activates the parasympathetic nervous system to establish homeostasis

    Exercise (aversive stimuli) activates enhanced mood, reduced anxiety, etc.

Physiological Explanations

4. Cerebral changes hypothesis (Cognitive functioning)

    a. Exercise produces structural changes including increased density of vasculature

    b. Increased blood flow during exercise provides increased nutrients (O^2 & glucose)

    Evidence does not seem to support = dose response unrelated to ES

END

Chapter 5: Physical Activity and Personality

The Psychology of Physical Activity
Albert V. Carron
Heather A. Hausenblas
Paul A. Estabrooks

**The self is not something ready-made,
but something in continuous formation
through choice of action**
John Dewey

**Can Personality be Changed through
Physical Activity?**

- Personality
  - Stable and enduring modifiable and dynamic aspects of the self

- Trait anxiety
- Self-esteem
- Body Image
- Social Physique Anxiety

1

Trait Anxiety and Physical Activity

🔔 Petruzzello et al. (1991) undertook a meta-analysis on studies examining the impact of physical activity on <u>trait anxiety</u>

🔔 An small overall effect size of .34

Trait Anxiety and Physical Activity: Moderators

🔔 Task type
  ➡ Aerobic activities slightly better than anaerobic but difference not statistically significant

🔔 Dose-response
  ➡ Minimal anxiety reductions before 9 weeks
  ➡ Large changes after 16 weeks
  ➡ Length of a session also important
  ➡ >20 min. related to increased anxiety

Perceptions of the Self

🔔 Self-concept
  ➡ The description of the self synonymous with personal identity e.g., "I am a regular exerciser"

🔔 Self-esteem
  ➡ The evaluation of the self synonymous with perceptions of self-worth e.g., "I am a good person"
  ➡ Theoreticians recognize that self-esteem is multidimensional

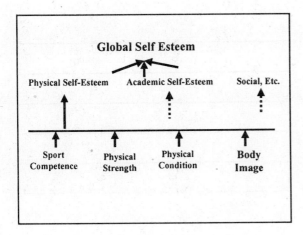

Global Self Esteem

Physical Self-Esteem   Academic Self-Esteem   Social, Etc.

Sport Competence   Physical Strength   Physical Condition   Body Image

---

Self-Esteem and Physical Activity

※ **The impact of activity on global self-esteem**

- ➡ Physical activity has a moderate effect on self-esteem (approx. .55)
- ➡ Physical activity does not automatically enhance self-esteem
- ➡ Greatest effects from exercise are for children and the elderly
- ➡ Dose-response studies show changes in self-esteem occur almost immediately

---

Physical Activity and Self-esteem

Children: 0.41
Young Adults: 0.55
Middle Adults: 0.57
Elderly: 0.61

■ Effect Size

Gruber, 1986; Hodges & McDonald, 1991

Body Image and Physical Activity

☼ **Internal view of your outer appearance**
  ➡ Cognitive
  ➡ Perceptual
  ➡ Behavioral
  ➡ Affective
  ➡ Subjective Evaluation

Thompson et al. (1999)

Body Dissatisfaction in Adults

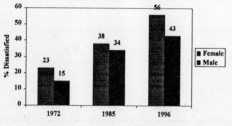

Berscheid et al. (1973); Garner (1997)

Body Image and Physical Activity

☼ **Meta-analysis--exercisers versus nonexercisers**
  ➡ ES=.29
  ➡ Exercisers have a more positive body image
☼ **Meta-analysis—experimental studies**
  ➡ ES=.15
  ➡ Physical activity had a small positive effect on body image.

Hausenblas & Fallon (2001)

Moderator: Type of Exercise

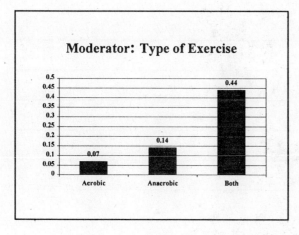

Physical Activity and Accurate Body Perceptions

- Perceptions of one's body shape and size are typically inaccurate

- Participation in regular physical activity improves the accuracy of self-perceptions regarding the body

Physical Activity and Anxiety About the Body

- Anxiety related to self-presentation

    → Self Presentation: Selective presentation of aspects of the self, omission of self-relevant information to maximize the likelihood that a positive social impression will be generated and an undesired impression will be avoided

Physical Activity and Anxiety About the Body

☼ **Social Physique Anxiety (SPA)**

- Social anxiety—concerns about the self-presentation of the body
- High SPA individuals often exercise for self-presentation reasons (e.g. to improve appearance)
- Regular physical activity has been shown to reduce SPA
- Being in groups with people one perceives as similar physically also reduces SPA.

END

_____

_____

_____

_____

_____

_____

_____

_____

_____

_____

_____

_____

Chapter 6: Psychobiological Benefits of
Physical Activity

The Psychology of Physical Activity
Albert V. Carron
Heather A. Hausenblas
Paul A. Estabrooks

**I have never taken any exercise except
sleeping and resting and I never intend
to take any.**
Mark Twain

**Psychobiological Benefits of Physical
Activity**

☼**Psychobiological Benefits**
➡ Sleep
➡ Reactivity to stressors
➡ Naturally occurring pain

Physical Activity and Sleep

🔔 **Insomnia influences 20-40% of world's population**

🔔 **Lack of sleep contributes to:**
- *Depression*
- *lack of productivity*
- *accidents (e.g., Chernobyl nuclear disaster)*

Physical Activity and Sleep

🔔 **Troubled sleep is often treated with sleeping medications**

🔔 **Medication (pills) problematic**
- Dependence problems
- Tolerance problems & rebound insomnia
- Pills health equivalent of smoking

🔔 **Self-reports suggest individuals believe regular physical activity may improve sleep**
- Validity problems with this research

Physical Activity and Sleep

🔔 **There have been a number of laboratory based studies that examine the relationship between sleep and physical activity**
- Muscle tension recordings
- EEG recordings
- EMG recordings

🔔 **To understand the results of these studies it is necessary to review the nature of sleep**

The Nature of Sleep

☼ **Stages:**
- Stage 1, 5% of total sleep--period between wakefulness & sleep
- Stage 2, 50%--reduced EEG activity
- Stage 3-4, 20%--minimal EEG activity "slow wave sleep" SWS
- REM, 25%--rapid eye-movement sleep

☼ **SWS (Stage 3-4 NREM) considered preferable for feelings of rejuvenation**

☼ **We move in and out of REM/NREM in 90 minute cycles**

Physical Activity and Sleep

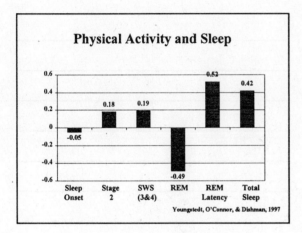

Youngstedt, O'Connor, & Dishman, 1997

Physical Activity and Sleep

☼ **Physical activity has a minimal impact on sleep but ...**
- Subjects in studies were healthy people without sleeping disorders
- No evidence that exercise immediately prior to bedtime disrupts sleep (NB. for practitioners!)
- Dose-response relationship is present: longer the exercise = longer total sleep time

3

Physical Activity and Reactivity to Stressors

☀ **Stress**
➜ Imbalance between demands (psychological or physical) and response capability

☀ **Examples of Biological Response to Stress:**
➜ Increased heart rate
➜ Increased respiratory rate
➜ Increased blood pressure

Physical Activity and Reactivity to Stressors

Crews & Landers, 1987

Possible Mechanisms?

1. **Coping hypothesis …**
   ➜ Physical activity produces a more efficient system so recovery of the Autonomic Nervous System (ANS) is quicker

2. **Inoculation hypothesis …**
   ➜ Chronic physical activity enhances our ability to handle stress
   ➜ Magnitude of response in well-trained systems is reduced

Physical Activity and Pain

- Pain is an unpleasant sensory and emotional experience associated with actual or potential tissue damage, or described in terms of such damage
    - A subjective experience
    - Emotions are an element
    - Not always related to tissue damage

- Pain causes functional impairment in 3-13% of the adult population

The Components of Pain

- Nocioeption
    - The detection of tissue damage by sensory receptors
- Perception of Pain
    - Experienced regardless of actual tissue damage
- Emotion
    - Unpleasantness, distress caused by pain
    - Cognitive appraisal of how pain will effect life
- Behavior
    - Activities performed or avoided as the result of pain

Physical Activity and Pain

- Physical activity has been effective in reducing naturally occurring pain in:
    - Individuals with Arthritis
    - Individuals with Fibromyalgia
    - Individuals with low back problems
    - Women during labor

Physical Activity and Pain

⚠ **Physical activity has been effective in:**

- ➡ Increasing the pain threshold immediately after and 15 minutes following an acute bout of physical activity
- ➡ Lower perceptions of the magnitude of pain following and acute bout of physical activity

---

END

_____

_____

_____

_____

_____

_____

_____

_____

_____

_____

_____

_____

Chapter 7: Negative Behaviors and Physical Activity

The Psychology of Physical Activity
Albert V. Carron
Heather A. Hausenblas
Paul A. Estabrooks

Every form of addiction is bad.
Carl Gustav Jung

Negative Behaviors and Physical Activity

☼ Can an activity associated with so many benefits have the potential to be harmful?
  ➡ Exercise dependence
  ➡ Physical activity and eating disorders
  ➡ Physical activity and steroid use

Exercise Dependence

※A number of definitions have been provided for exercise dependence that include:

    (a) Behavioral correlates that might reflect dependence including physical activity duration, intensity, and/or frequency

    (b) Psychological correlates that might reflect dependence including a pathological commitment to PA

    (c) A combination of both

※There are thousands of people who can be physically active 5, 6, or even 7 days a week who may not be exercise dependent

---

Exercise Dependence

※Dependence is indicated not only by the behavior but by the psychological reasons underlying that behavior

※David Veale (1987;1995) advocated the adoption of a set of standards for diagnosing exercise dependence that are based on the Diagnostic and Statistical Manual for Mental Disorders criteria for substance dependence (DSM; American Psychiatric Association [APA], 1994)

Exercise Dependence

※Exercise dependence can be defined as a multidimensional maladaptive pattern of PA, leading to significant impairment or distress, as manifested by three or more criteria from a possible list of seven.

Exercise Dependence

☼ **The seven criteria are:**

1) <u>Tolerance</u> effects--either increased amounts of PA are required to achieve the desired effect or the individual experiences markedly diminished effects from the same amount of PA

2) <u>Withdrawal</u> effects -- either symptoms such as anxiety or fatigue are evidenced with cessation of PA or PA is used to relieve or forestall the onset of the symptoms

3) <u>Intention</u> effects -- PA is undertaken with greater intensity, frequency, or duration than was intended

---

Exercise Dependence

☼ **The seven criteria are:**

4) <u>Lack of control</u> -- PA is maintained despite a persistent desire to cut down or control it

5) <u>Time</u> -- considerable time is spent in activities essential to PA maintenance

6) <u>Reduction in other activities</u> -- other social, occupational, or recreational pursuits are reduced or dropped because of PA

7) <u>Continuance</u> -- despite the awareness of a persistent physical or psychological problem, PA is maintained; e.g., running in spite of shin splints)

Historical Contributions

☼**Frederick Baekeland in 1970**

➡ First, he couldn't recruiting habitual male exercisers willing to abstain from PA for one month

➡ Second, during the one month deprivation period in the study, participants began to report decreased psychological well-being

☼**Difference between positive and negative addiction?**

3

Exercise Dependence Research

☼ A recent review, concluded that the exercise dependence research is characterized by three general approaches:
- ➡ Comparing exercisers to eating disorder patients
- ➡ Comparing "excessive" to "less excessive" exercisers
- ➡ Comparing exercisers to nonexercisers

Exercise Dependence Research

☼ Limitations of this research
- ➡ Lack of experimental investigations
- ➡ Inconsistent or nonexistent control groups
- ➡ Failure to control for subject biases
- ➡ Discrepant classification criteria, and/or invalid or inappropriate measures for excessive dependence

---

Recent Exercise Dependence Research

☼ Hausenblas and Symons (in press) examined exercise dependence in over 2,300 exercisers who varied in their involvement.
- ➡ 9% of the exercisers could be classified as exercise dependent
- ➡ 40% as nondependent-symptomatic
- ➡ 41% as nondependent-asymptomatic

Exercise Deprivation

🔔 **Represent effects during periods of no physical activity**

🔔 **Symptoms:**
- ➡ Affective: i.e., anxiety, depression
- ➡ Cognitive: i.e., confusion, concentration
- ➡ Physiological: i.e., fatigue, sleep
- ➡ Social: i.e., increased social interaction

Consequences of Deprivation in Habitual Exercisers

🔔 **Mondin et al. (1996)**

🔔 **Purpose:**
- ➡ Evaluate the influence of 3 day exercise deprivation on psychological variables

🔔 **Participants**
- ➡ 10 male and female habitual runners
- ➡ M age = 27
- ➡ Exercised 6/7 days a week for 45 min.

Measures

🔔 **Profile of Mood States (POMS):**
- ➡ tension, vigor (positive), depression, anger, fatigue, confusion

🔔 **State-Trait Anxiety Inventory**
- ➡ Spielberger et al. (1983)

🔔 **Depression Adjective Checklist**
- ➡ Lubin et al. (1978)

Procedure

- 5 day study

- Monday & Friday (exercise days)
  - ➡ completed psychological measures

- Tues & Wed & Thurs (no exercise)
  - ➡ completed psychological measures

Results

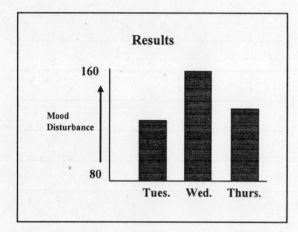

- 3 days of exercise deprivation resulted in increases in:
  - ➡ Total mood disturbance
  - ➡ State anxiety
  - ➡ Depression
- Resumed exercise resulted in:
  - ➡ Mood improvement

Explanations of Exercise Dependence

- Psychological
  - Personality Trait Explanation
  - Anorexia Analogue Hypothesis
  - Affective Regulation explanation

- Physiological
  - β-endorphin Explanation
  - Sympathetic Arousal Explanation

- Psychobiological Explanations
  - Subjective Aversion

Treatment of Exercise Dependence

- Adams & Kirkby (1997) interviewed 24 physiotherapists w/ exercise-dependent clients.
- Treatments:
  a) Educate about injury and likely outcomes
  b) Prescribe reduced or alternative activities
  c) Refer to other health professionals
  d) Use psychological strategies, i.e., behavior modification, modeling, and counseling.

- 71% physiotherapists experienced problems communicating -- the injured runners simply refused to stop exercising .

Over Training and Staleness

- Over training
  - Short period of training during which people increase their training loads to near or to maximal capacity
  - Anorexia Analogue Hypothesis
  - Affective Regulation explanation

- Over training may lead to staleness
  - A psychological state that manifests as deteriorated readiness
  - Impairment of performance
  - Increased depression

Physical Activity and Eating Disorders

- Individuals often have unrealistic expectations related to weight management and PA.

- Images of the ideal body
  - thin and fit for women
  - fit and muscular for men

- Diet is often used to attempt to model these ideals.

Anorexia Nervosa

1. Refusal to maintain body weight at or above a minimally normal weight for age and height

2. Intense fear of gaining weight or becoming fat, even though under weight

3. Disturbance in the way in which one's body weight or shape is experienced, unduly influence of body weight or shape on self-evaluation, or denial of the seriousness of the current low body weight

4. Amenorrhea

Bulimia Nervosa

1. Recurrent episodes of binge eating.
   a) a discrete period=more food than most people
   b) a sense of lack of control over eating during the episode

2. Recurrent inappropriate compensatory behavior in order to prevent weight gain

3. The binge eating and inappropriate compensatory behaviors both occur, on average, at least twice a week for three months

4. Self-evaluation is unduly influenced by body shape and weight

5. The disturbance does not occur exclusively during episodes of anorexia nervosa

Physical Activity and Eating Disorders

- If progress in weight management seems slow compulsive exercise may be added to speed up weight loss

- The relationship between PA and eating disorders is not clear

- Some experts have stated that there is no relationship between PA and eating disorders

- Other experts feel that there is.

Eating Disorders versus Excessive Physical Activity

- Is exercise dependence a variant of anorexia nervosa?
  - Eating disorder diagnosis must first be excluded before a diagnosis of primary exercise dependence can be made.

- Primary exercise dependence= PA is an end in itself

- Secondary exercise dependence=the motivation for PA is the control and manipulation of body composition.

Eating Disorder Patients versus Excessive Physical Activity

- Examination of physical activity as a manifestation of anorexia nervosa.

- Alayne Yates and her colleagues (1983) who argued that male obligatory runners resembled anorexia nervosa

- Were introverted, did not display anger, had high expectations, were depressed, and were in denial

- Heavily criticized--lack of data, poor methods, overstated similarities between the groups.

Eating Disorder Patients versus Excessive Physical Activity

- Subsequent controlled studies have compared eating disorder patients and exercisers have yielded conflicting results.

- Robust psychological similarities between eating disordered individuals and exercisers have not been identified

---

Eating Disorder Patients versus Excessive Physical Activity

- Powers and her colleagues (1998) examined psychological and physiological characteristics of 40 male and female obligatory runners and 17 female anorexia nervosa patients.
  - The runners: (a) ran over 25 miles/week, (b) ran despite injury or illness, (c) considered running to be an important part of their life, and (d) felt guilty, irritable, or depressed when unable to run
- Measures of depression, personality, obsessions, body image, body composition, and fitness were obtained.

Eating Disorder Patients versus Excessive Physical Activity

- Anorexia nervosa patients displayed significant psychopathology

- Runners were consistently in the normal range

- Body fat was in the normal range for the runners and low in the anorexia nervosa group

- Runners had excellent fitness levels compared to the anorexia nervosa patients

- Those with anorexia nervosa and habitual runners did not possess similar psychological or physiological features

Comparison of Athletes to Nonathletes

☼ **Athletes as a population might be at-risk**

  1) Societal norms --favor a lean physically fit physique -- these societal norms are salient for athletes

  2) High activity levels and strenuous exercise can reduce the value of food reinforcement

  3) Psychological characteristics consistent with high-level athletic achievement (perfectionism, motivation), are also evident in individuals with eating disorders

☼ **It does appear that athletes as a population self-report more eating disorder symptoms than do nonathletes.**

Comparison of Athletes to Nonathletes

☼ **Hausenblas and Carron (1999) meta-analysis**

  ➡ Female athletes self-reported more bulimic (ES = .16) and anorexic (ES = .12) symptoms compared to females from the general population

  ➡ Male athletes self-reported more bulimic (ES = .30) and anorexic (ES = .35) symptoms compared to males from the general population.

Comparison of Athletes to Nonathletes

☼ **Hausenblas and Carron (1999) meta-analysis**

  ➡ Male athletes in aesthetic and weight-dependent sports self-reported more bulimic and drive for thinness symptomatology versus male comparison groups.

  ➡ Females in aesthetic sports self-reported more of the tendencies to report anorexic symptoms (ES = .38)

Steroid Abuse and Physical Activity

☼Steroids-- man-made versions of the primary male sex hormone, testosterone

☼Athletes are not the only population using steroids.
  ➡Fireman
  ➡Policemen
  ➡Military personnel
  ➡Personal trainers
  ➡Regular exercisers

Steroid Abuse and Physical Activity

☼How prevalent is steroid use?

  ➡The first nationwide survey of steroid use among teenage boys 1988
  ➡About 7% of high school seniors had used steroids.
  ➡Prevalent in wrestling and football
  ➡35% of steroid users did not participate in any sport

Steroid Abuse and Physical Activity

☼Reasons for use
  ➡Improve athletic performance (47%)
  ➡Improve physical appearance (27%)
  ➡Prevent or treat injury (11%)
  ➡Fit in (7%)

☼The results of the Buckely et al. (1988) study subsequently have been confirmed by more than 40 national, regional, and local studies

Steroid Abuse and Physical Activity

☼ Pope & Katz (1994) examined the psychological effects of steroid use

☼ Urine samples were obtained to assess actual steroid use.

☼ 23% reported experiencing major mood disturbances (i.e., mania, anxiety, depression, or major depression).

Muscle Dsymorphia

☼ A large variety of terms have been used to describe a form of body image distortion in which the individual perceives him/herself as unacceptably small.
   (a) pathologically preoccupied with the appearance of the whole body
   (b) concerned that they are not sufficiently large or muscular
   (c) are consumed by weightlifting, dieting, and steroid abuse.

END

Chapter 8: Individual Correlates of Physical Activity

The Psychology of Physical Activity
Albert V. Carron
Heather A. Hausenblas
Paul A. Estabrooks

If a man would move the world, he
must first move himself.
Socrates

Individual Correlates of Physical Activity

- ✿ 30 min. daily of moderate intensity PA
- ✿ Moderate intensity?? ……
  - ➡ Walking at a pace of 3-4 miles per hr.
  - ➡ Moderate intensity activities positively associated with adherence
- ✿ High intensity negatively related to adherence
- ✿ But … benefits are related to intensity and duration

OTHER CONSIDERATIONS

🔔 **For some people frequent bouts of shorter duration may be beneficial**

🔔 **Jackicic et al. (1995) ...... 56 overweight adult females exercised**
  - ➤ Weeks 1-4 .... 20 min/day
  - ➤ Weeks 5-8 ..... 30 min/day
  - ➤ Weeks 9-20 .... 40 min/day

🔔 **Long bout group = 1 exercise period**

🔔 **Short bout group = 10 min blocks**

🔔 **Found adherence (days & duration/day) better in short bout**

Individual Correlates of Physical Activity

🔔 **To promote regular physical activity it is important to gain insight into the factors associated with physical activity**

🔔 **Correlation versus causation; e.g. income**

🔔 **Over 300 studies have examined the correlates of physical activity** (Sallis & Owen, 1998)

Demographic & Biological Correlates of PA

🔔 **Age**
🔔 **Gender**
🔔 **Ethnicity**
🔔 **Occupation**
🔔 **Education level**
🔔 **Health status**

Demographic & Biological Correlates of PA

☼ **These types of characteristics cannot be altered.**

☼ **Why is it important to study them?**

➡ To identify groups more at-risk for inactivity

➡ To target specific intervention strategies for different populations.

Age

☼ **Physical activity decline with age ....**
➡ an almost 50% decrease between ages 6 and 16

☼ **Physical activity also decreases from adulthood to older adulthood .... why?**

☼ **Advancing age is associated with**
➡ Reductions in cardiovascular fitness
➡ Impaired health (e.g., arthritis)
➡ Retirement
➡ Isolation from others due to poor health

Gender

☼ **Gender differences in the physical activity patterns of infants are minimal.**

☼ **At all other ages males engage in more vigorous and moderate physical active than females.**

Ethnicity

⚜ **Surveys and epidemiological studies have found that ethnic differences exist for sedentariness.**

- ➡ 36% of White or Caucasian Americans are sedentary
- ➡ 42% of Asian or Pacific Islanders
- ➡ 46% of American Pacific Islanders,
- ➡ 52% of African Americans,
- ➡ 54% of Hispanic Americans

Occupation & Education Level

⚜ **Blue-collar workers are less likely to ....**
- ➡ participate in leisure-time physical activity
- ➡ use worksite exercise facilities
- ➡ stay in rehabilitative exercise programs following myocardial infarction

⚜ **Level of education is positively associated with leisure-time physical activity:**
- ➡ < 9th grade education = 6% of adults
- ➡ >= college degree = 32% of adults

Education Level

Parental education level is related to child physical activity

Parent's Education	% Active
At least 1 yr. University	68%
High school graduate	54%
LT high school	50%

Education Level of Others

- People who live in neighborhoods where many neighbors hold college degrees are more likely to walk.

- Is this an impact of education?
  - Results provide evidence for a contagion effect, behaviors seen in neighborhood are adopted

Biomedical Status

- Physical activity is less in ....
  - unhealthy vs. healthy people
  - obese vs. normal weight
  - people with disabilities (13%)

- Injury
  - Regular exercisers are more likely to report injuries (Sallis, et. Al., 1990)

Psychological Correlates

- Negatively associated with PA
  - Perceived barriers
  - Mood disturbances
- Positively associated with PA
  - Enjoyment
  - Perceived fitness or health
  - Self-efficacy
  - Self-schemata
- Not associated with PA
  - Perceived susceptibility to illness
  - Knowledge

Enjoyment

☼ People who enjoy PA are more active

☼ Sallis et al. (1999) examined 22 potential determinants of PA in 1,504 children in grades 4 to 12 ....
  ➡ Enjoyment one of the strongest determinants of PA.

☼ Causes or Effects?

Characteristics of Physical Activity

☼ Intensity & Perceived Effort
  ➡ Higher the perceived effort and intensity of PA, the less likely people are to adhere

☼ Duration
  ➡ Long-bout vs. short-bout

Behavioral Correlates of Physical Activity

☼ Smoking
☼ Diet
☼ Previous PA history

Smoking

- Negative relationship between cigarette smoking and PA
  - Relatively modest relationship.
  - Some studies show no association
  - Others show smoking related to higher dropout rates from vigorous activity programs

Diet

- Eating frequency negatively related to PA

- Milk intake negatively related PA

- In general, good dietary habits are positively correlated with PA

History Of Physical Activity

- Tracking--children maintaining their relative ranking on a variable over time

- Tracking in Physical Activity--childhood to adolescence to adulthood

END

8

Chapter 9: Physical Activity Groups

The Psychology of Physical Activity
Albert V. Carron
Heather A. Hausenblas
Paul A. Estabrooks

Those who are enjoying something, or suffering something, together, are companions.
C.S. Lewis

Group Dynamics And Physical Activity

The importance of group dynamics in physical activity promotion is its ability to identify:

➡ The forces that bind members to their groups
➡ The critical parameters of leadership
➡ The impact of group structure

Group Dynamics And Physical Activity

🔔 Forces that Bind Members to Their Groups: Class Cohesion

🔔 A dynamic process that is reflected in the tendency for a group to stick together and remain united in pursuit of its instrumental objectives and/or for the satisfaction of member affective needs

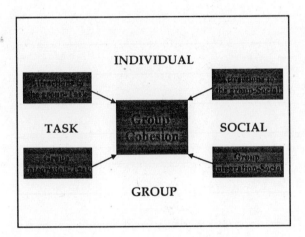

INDIVIDUAL

Attractions to the group-Task

Attractions to the group-Social

TASK   Group Cohesion   SOCIAL

Group integration-Task

Group integration-Social

GROUP

The Measurement of Cohesion

🔔 The Measurement of Cohesion in Physical Activity Classes

➡ The Group Environment Questionnaire (GEQ)
➡ Physical Activity Group Environment Questionnaire (PAGEQ)

Cohesion and Adherence Behavior

🔔 **Carron, Widmeyer, and Brawley (1988)**

- First to show that physical activity program adherers and dropouts differed in their perceptions of cohesion
- Adherers had higher perceptions of ATGT and ATGS

Cohesion and Adherence Behavior

🔔 **Spink and Carron (1992)**

- Females participating in exercise classes
- 4 weeks of attendance and punctuality data were collected during Weeks 8 to 12 of a 13-week program
- GEQ at Week 13
- ATGT and ATGS, were negatively associated with absenteeism
- ATGT accounted for the greatest difference between those participants who were never late and those who were late four or more times.

Cohesion and Adherence Behavior

🔔 Previous studies were retrospective in nature...

🔔 Spink and Carron conducted two prospective studies to examine the predictive ability of group cohesion for exercise adherence

- Study 1 --GEQ in Week 3 of a 13-week program university fitness class
- Attendance during the final 4 weeks
- Dropouts from the 13-week program had possessed lower perceptions of ATGT than the adherers

Cohesion and Adherence Behavior

☼Spink and Carron Study 2--a private fitness facility rather than in a university setting

- ➡ GEQ --3rd week of a 13-week program
- ➡ Attendance again was monitored for the final four weeks of the program
- ➡ Dropouts had lower perceptions ATGS and GIS

Cohesion and Adherence Behavior

☼Initial research with younger adults
☼Important to look at older adults?

- ➡ Aging has a deleterious effect
- ➡ PA is positively associated with physical and psychological maintenance and improvements for older adults
- ➡ If a group and/or the presence of high cohesion are found to be beneficial for older adults, important implications are present for program planning.

Cohesion and Adherence Behavior

☼Estabrooks and Carron (1999) examined the relationship between class cohesion and exercise adherence in older adults

- ➡ Study 1, 14 exercise classes for older adults completed the GEQ during the first month of a new exercise term
- ➡ Attendance at the program was then documented for 1, 6, and 12 months
- ➡ ATGS, GIS, and GIT at one-month interval
- ➡ GIT was significantly related to class attendance following a 6- and 12-month interval

Cohesion and Adherence Behavior

☆ Given the consistent findings of these studies and others it has been concluded that the relationship between group cohesion and exercise adherence exists.

☆ Why?
  ➔ Group processes
  ➔ Individual mechanisms

_____

_____

_____

_____

_____

_____

Group Cohesion And Group Processes

☆ Hill and Estabrooks (2000) studied the relationship between group cohesion and group interaction

  ➔ Competitiveness was positively associated with ATGT and GIT
  ➔ Communication had the strongest positive relationship ATGS
  ➔ Competition, cooperation, and communication were positively related to GIS

_____

_____

_____

_____

_____

_____

Group Cohesion And Individual Cognitions

☆ Perceptions of control positively related to ATGT (Estabrooks & Carron, 1999).

☆ Self-efficacy to schedule physical activity classes into one's regular routine positively related to ATGT & GIT (Estabrooks & Carron, 2000)

☆ ATGT, ATGS, & GIT were positively associated with affect (Courneya, 1995)

☆ ATGT & ATGS were positively related to attitude (Estabrooks & Carron, 1999)

_____

_____

_____

_____

_____

_____

Leadership And Physical Activity

🔔Researchers and program planners also have been interested in the role that exercise leaders play in participants' attitudes toward and adherence in PA programs

🔔Oldridge (1977) concluded that the exercise leader is "the pivot on which the success or failure of a program will depend"

Leadership And Physical Activity

🔔Franklin (1988) compiled a list of over 30 variables that influence dropout behaviour from physical activity programs, he identified the exercise leader as "the single most important variable affecting exercise compliance"

🔔Carron, Hausenblas, and Mack (1996) Meta-analysis
  ➡ A small effect for the influence that class leaders have on adherence behavior.

Leadership And Physical Activity

🔔Susan Peterson (1993) identified 24 qualities that can be reduced to three general categories—behavioral, communicative and motivational.

  ➡ Behavioral--the ability to instruct with the proper technical execution, stay focused, and be energetic.
  ➡ Communicative--Class leaders should possess the ability to express themselves clearly and listen to class members.
  ➡ Motivational--leaders should have the ability to motivate both the participants and themselves, be decisive, and use group processes.

Leadership And Physical Activity

☼ **McAuley and Jacobson (1991)**
- ➡ Following an 8-week program, participants were asked how they felt their instructor had influenced their adherence to the program
- ➡ Participant perceptions of leader influence did have a small positive association with in-class adherence

☼ **Nancy Gyurcsik and her associates (1998)**
- ➡ Assessed participants' confidence in their activity leader's abilities
- ➡ Monitored attendance for 12 weeks
- ➡ A small, but significant, relationship was found with attendance

Leadership And PA Participation

☼ **Fox and her collaborators (2000) investigated the impact of leadership style and group dynamics on intention to return to a structured fitness class**

- ➡ Manipulated leadership style (i.e., an enriched versus a bland leadership style)
- ➡ Manipulated the group environment (i.e., an enriched versus a bland class environment) were systematically varied.

Leadership And Physical Activity

☼ The enriched group environment was manipulated with the use of trained confederates

☼ Intention to return to a similar class and enjoyment of the session was assessed

☼ Enriched leadership & group environment= Increased enjoyment

☼ Those in the enriched group environments intended to return to a similar exercise session, regardless of the style of the leader

Leadership And Physical Activity

❊Earlier in this section, it was noted that the physical activity class leader has been identified as possibly the most important factor in participant adherence.

❊However, research has not supported this contention

❊Only a small to moderate effect (ES = .31) is present for class leaders and adherence
(Carron et al., 1996)

Leadership And Physical Activity

❊Possible explanations for contradictory perspectives:

➡ First, the quotes by Oldridge and Franklin introduced in the first paragraph of this section, were broad statements of impact unburdened by data

➡ Second, most research on physical activity leadership compares the standard care (i.e., a regular instructor) to a special treatment

➡ Third, it is possible that the relationship between a class leader's behavior and the adherence of group members is small

---

Leadership And Physical Activity

❊It is possible that different or inadequate criteria (measurement, manipulations) were used to represent leadership in the physical activity domain

❊Within general leadership theory literature, research has "been regarded as a fractured and confusing set of contradictory findings and assertions without coherence or interpretability" (Chemers, 2000)

Group Size And Physical Activity

☼ **In a study focusing on adherence behavior**
(Carron et al., 1990, Study 1)

☼ **Examined archival data from 47 university physical activity classes**

☼ **Size ranged from 5-46 members**

☼ **Classes were classified as:**
- ➡ small classes (5 to 17 members)
- ➡ medium classes (18-26)
- ➡ moderately large classes (37-31)
- ➡ large classes (32-46)

Group Size And Physical Activity

☼ **Small and large classes had the highest retention rates (i.e., fewest dropouts) and superior attendance (i.e., percentage of classes attended by adherers)**

Group Size And Individual Perceptions

☼ **Research outside of the physical activity sciences shows that increasing group size generally has negative effects on group member perceptions** (Carron & Hausenblas, 1998)

☼ **Increasing group size:**
- ➡ more resources
- ➡ chances of meeting attractive and interesting others increases

☼ **However, across most types of groups generally see little positive benefit in increases in group size**

Group Size And Individual Perceptions

- ☼ **What about physical activity classes? Is the issue of group size relevant?**

- ☼ **Carron and his associates (1990) assessed the relationship between group size and...**
  - ➡ Member perceptions their leader
  - ➡ Crowding
  - ➡ Opportunities for interaction
  - ➡ Density
  - ➡ Satisfaction with the group

Group Size And Individual Perceptions

- ☼ **As physical activity classes became larger:**

  - ➡ participant perceptions of the instructor decreased in a linear fashion
  - ➡ participants in small and moderate sized classes perceived that more opportunities were available for social interaction than did those in large classes
  - ➡ Participants' satisfaction decreased in a linear fashion as class size increased from small to large

Group Size And Group Cohesion

- ☼ **The relationship between class size and perceptions of cohesion has also been examined**

- ☼ **Group Integration-Task and Social was lower in large classes** (Carron & Spink, 1995, Study 1)

- ☼ **Only when group cohesion was assessed late in the program**

Group Size And Group Cohesion

🔔 When cohesion was assessed earlier Individual Attractions to the Group-Task was lower in larger classes (Carron & Spink, 1995, Study 2)

🔔 In sum, the studies showed that members of small physical activity classes held stronger perceptions of cohesion than members of large classes

END

_____

_____

_____

_____

_____

_____

_____

_____

_____

_____

_____

_____

11

Chapter 10: Social Support and Physical Activity

The Psychology of Physical Activity
Albert V. Carron
Heather A. Hausenblas
Paul A. Estabrooks

Cherish your human connections, your relationships with friends and families
Barbara Bush

Social Support and Physical Activity

- What is Social Support
- Importance of Social Support to Health
- Shortcomings in the Assessment of Social Support in Research
- Why/How does Social Support Work?

What is Social Support?

☼ **Complex construct as indicated by...**
- ➡ Variety of definitions
- ➡ Variety of terms
- ➡ Variety of manifestations
- ➡ Relationship to personality

Definitions of Social Support

☼ **Information perspective:**
- ➡ Social support is information that causes person to feel cared for loved, and a sense of belonging

☼ **Emotion perspective:**
- ➡ Social support represents the gratification of a person's needs

Definitions of Social Support

☼ **Process perspective:**
- ➡ Social support is a dynamic process involving transactions between individuals

☼ **Network perspective :**
- ➡ Person is seen as focus of networks that vary in structure, linkages, functions

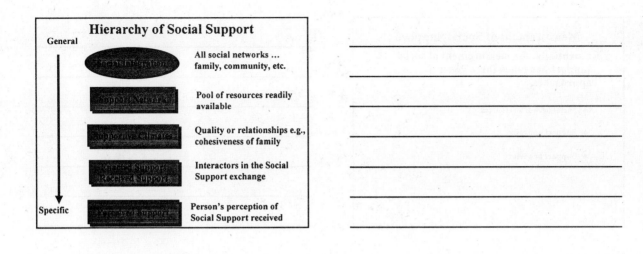

Hierarchy of Social Support

General

All social networks ... family, community, etc.

Pool of resources readily available

Quality or relationships e.g., cohesiveness of family

Interactors in the Social Support exchange

Specific

Person's perception of Social Support received

Negative & Personality Aspects of Social Support

☼ Social Support can also be negative :
  ➜ Social rejection or social hindrance

☼ Negative Social Support occurs infrequently:
  ➜ Likely has greater impact on physical activity
  ➜ e.g. "you might injure yourself"

☼ Social Support as a Personality Trait:
  ➜ People differ in the degree to which they feel supported, esteemed, loved
  ➜ Associated with self-esteem, self-concept

Measurement of Social Support

☼ How should social support be measured?

☼ Given the complex nature of social support, a number of approaches have been taken in its measurement

☼ Who gives the person social support?

☼ What type(s) of social support does an individual receive?

☼ What is the quantity and quality of that social support?

Measurement of Social Support

☼ Essentially, the measurement of social support has taken three general approaches

- ➡ Social network resources
- ➡ Support appraisal
- ➡ Support behavior

Measurement of Social Support

☼ Support appraisal
- ➡ Attachment—emotional support
- ➡ Social integration—network support
- ➡ Opportunity for nurturance—increased self worth from assisting others
- ➡ Reassurance of worth—esteem support
- ➡ Reliable alliance—tangible aid
- ➡ Guidance—information support

☼ Support behavior
- ➡ The focus is on <u>frequency of occurrence</u> or the <u>likelihood</u> that others will provide support

Social Support and Physical Activity

☼ In a recent meta-analysis the general role of social support in physical activity participation was examined

- ➡ The effect size of social support on adherence is in the small to moderate range
- ➡ The effect size of social support on the intention to be physically active is moderate

Social Support and Physical Activity

🔔 Adherence behavior is more strongly influenced by social support from important others than from family members

🔔 Recall:
  ➡ Adherence = maintaining involvement in a self-selected program
  ➡ Compliance = maintaining involvement in a prescribed program

🔔 In compliance social support from family plays an important role (ES=.69)

Social Support and Cognitions

🔔 Research reported by Terry Duncan and his colleagues (Duncan & McAuley, 1993; Duncan & Stoolmiller, 1993) offers insight into how social support might play a role in involvement in physical activity

🔔 They found that both barriers and exercise efficacy served as a mediator between social support and physical activity

🔔 Social support contributes directly to efficacy which in turn contributes directly to physical activity behavior

---

Social Support and Cognitions

🔔 Social support has also been related to other physical activity related variables

🔔 Estabrooks and Carron (2000) also found that cohesion was related to social support

🔔 Task cohesion was related to reliable alliance and guidance

🔔 Social cohesion was related to reassurance of worth and attachment

Social Support and Cognitions

☼Courneya and McAuley (1995) examined the relationships between social support and subjective norm

➡ Subjective norm = the perceived social pressure to perform or not to perform the behavior" (Ajzen, 1991, p. 188)

➡ Found average correlations of .06, .20, and .30 over the three time periods that they tested.

Social Support and Mortality

Hanson et al. (1989) examined the relationship between all-cause mortality and

ocial networks

ocial support

Social influence

☼ Method Random sample of 50% of

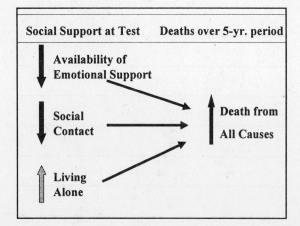

Social Support at Test   Deaths over 5-yr. period

Availability of Emotional Support

Social Contact → Death from All Causes

Living Alone

Social Support and Mortality

Blazer (1982)

ocial support in a elderly population
assessed & mortality determined 30 mo.

he elderly with greatest risk of dying
were those with

owest perceived social support

END

Chapter 11: Environmental Correlates of
Physical Activity

The Psychology of Physical Activity
Albert V. Carron
Heather A. Hausenblas
Paul A. Estabrooks

**The physical jerks would begin in three
minutes… "Smith!" screamed the
shrewish voice from the telescreen.
"6079 Smith W! Yes You! Bend lower,
please!"**
George Orwell

Environment And Physical Activity

☼ The introductory quote is from George
Orwell's novel '1984'

☼ In Big Brother's world there were no
adherence problems--100% prevalence,
100% maintenance.

☼ So, did Orwell, find the answer to
promoting the initiation and maintenance of
physical activity?

Environment And Physical Activity

※One's environment has the potential to be related to behavioral outcomes

※A functional starting point is with Walter Mischel and his associates' research regarding delayed gratification in children
- Children were shown toys, marshmallows, or candies.
- Have it now, or have more later
- Left alone for 20 minutes

Environment and Physical Activity

※The children, on average, were not very successful in delaying their gratification-- most would quickly play with the toys or eat the candies.

※However, there were some children who could wait until the researchers returned (Mischel, Shoda, & Rodriguez, 1989)

※Why could some children control themselves and wait, while others hardly blinked before consuming candy?

Environment and Physical Activity

※Taught half the children to think about fun thoughts while waiting for the researcher to return.
- Condition 1 the children were asked to wait while the candy was in plain view on the table
- Condition 2, the children were asked to wait while the candy was on the table but under a cover.

Think Fun: Delay Time in Minutes

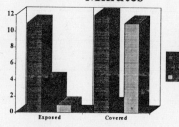

Approximate data from Mischel et al., (1972)

Environment And Physical Activity

☼ How does this related to physical activity participation?

➡ First, like waiting for a second candy, the benefits of physical activity participation are sometimes more distal than the acute benefits of sedentary behaviors.

➡ Second, like waiting for candy, physical activity often takes coping skills to complete.

Environment And Physical Activity

☼ It can be concluded that when the environment is risky (i.e., there is a candy waiting to be eaten or a television show waiting to be watched), it is important to ensure that individuals have appropriate coping skills

☼ When the environment is supportive (i.e., no candy, accessible physical activity options), even those people without appropriate coping skills can be successful.

The Western Environment

🔔 Rode & Shephard (1994) studied the effects of modernization in a community of Canadian Inuit

🔔 In 1970, before acculturation, both Inuit men and women were more aerobically fit than age-matched men in industrialized nations, but by 1990, the Inuit physical superiority had become much less pronounced

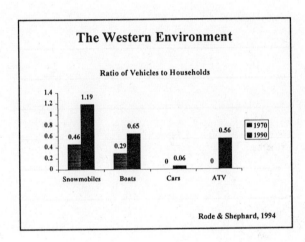

The Western Environment

Ratio of Vehicles to Households

Rode & Shephard, 1994

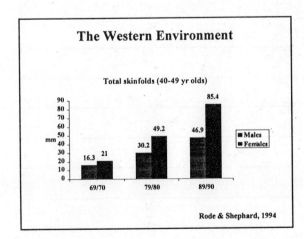

The Western Environment

Total skinfolds (40-49 yr olds)

Rode & Shephard, 1994

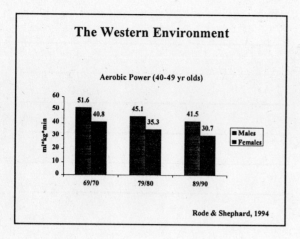

The Western Environment

Aerobic Power (40-49 yr olds)

- Males
- Females

Rode & Shephard, 1994

Environment And Physical Activity

☼ Travel patterns of people from different industrialized countries

☼ Netherlands

→ Trips of one kilometer or less --32% and 60% were traveled by bicycle and walking respectively

→ Trips of covering distances between 1 and 2.5 kilometers 46% and 21% were traveled by bicycle and walking respectively

→ Transportation by car only accounted for 44% of all trips within urban areas

---

Environment And Physical Activity

☼ North American countries have very low bicycle and walking patterns within urban areas

☼ Canadians only use a bicycle for 1% of all trips, and walk for 10%, and travel by car for 74% of all trips

☼ Americans travel by car 84% of all urban trips, bicycle for 1%, and walk for 9% (Pucher & Lefevre, 1996)

Environment And Physical Activity

☼☀One factor that may account for the differences between these populations is the the road system (Pucher & Lefevre, 1996)

☼☀Netherlands--urban roads and paths are made to facilitate cycling and walking.
  ➡ Right of way and separate lanes are provided for cyclists

☼☀North America--many urban communities are developed without sidewalks and clearly with car travel in mind (Pucher & Lefevre, 1996)

Environment And Physical Activity

☼☀It could be argued that it is cultural norms that really affect the travel patterns of populations in the Netherlands, United States, and Canada

☼☀Although, cultural norms undoubtedly have some impact on travel patterns, studies in both the United States and Canada have shown that 46% and 70% of respondents respectively, would cycle to work more often if safe bicycle lanes were provided

Environment And Physical Activity

☼☀In 1985, Rod Dishman and his associates categorized the determinants into personal characteristics and environmental influences.

☼☀The weather, distance from facilities, and time pressures were all considered to be influences of one's environment.

Environment And Physical Activity

- ☼ Donald Iverson and his colleagues reviewed research examining physical activity promotion in medical, worksite, community, and school settings.

- ☼ Concluded:
  - ➡ Less active individuals would become more active if facilities were more accessible, of better quality, and cheaper
  - ➡ Community environmental changes such as building bicycle paths, walking trails, basketball courts, and swimming pools should increase physical activity.

Environmental Prompts

- ☼ Brownell, Stunkard, and Albaum (1980; Study 1) provided the seminal study on the potential impact of one's environment on subsequent physical activity
- ☼ Placed a sign at the stairs/escalator choice point
  - ➡ The sign was three by three and a half feet and depicted a lethargic heavy heart riding up the escalator and a healthy slim heart climbing the stairs
- ☼ Stair use increased from 5-6% up to 13-16%

Perceived Access

- ☼ Sallis et al. (1997) had undergraduates indicate physical activity resources available to them
- ☼ Home environment; e.g., equipment
- ☼ Neighborhood environment
  - ➡ Features; e.g. bike paths
  - ➡ Perceived safety
  - ➡ Type of environment; e.g., residential, commercial
- ☼ Convenience to 18 types of facilities
- ☼ Physical activity was assessed

Perceived Access

Sallis et al. found:

- The perceived home environment was related to physical activity.
- The perceived neighborhood environment was NOT related to physical activity
- The perceived convenience of facilities had a small relationship to PA

Perceived Access

Booth et al. (2000) had adults <60 years indicate physical activity resources available to them

Home environment

Neighborhood environment

- Features
- Perceived safety
- Access to facilities

2 Week recall of physical activity obtained

Perceived Access

Booth et al. found:

- The perceived home environment was NOT related to physical activity.
- The perceived neighborhood environment was NOT related to physical activity
- The perceived access to facilities was related to physical activity

Actual Access to Resources

- Sallis et al. (1990) phoned a random sample of 2053 residents of San Diego
- Physical activity levels determined
- Address obtained (to match against address of local facilities)
- PA of each respondent matched with density of facilities in his/her neighborhoods
- They found that the density of neighborhood facilities was related to physical activity

What about the issue of access?

- Estabrooks, Lee, & Gyurcsik (in press) investigated the availability accessibility of physical activity resources with a small mid-western city

- A secondary purpose was to examine community socioeconomic status in relation to the identified physical activity resources

Neighborhood Context and Physical Activity

Data source: Yen, I.H., & Kaplan, G.A. (1998). Poverty area residence and changes in physical activity level: Evidence from the Alameda County Study. *AJPH, 88*, 1709-1712.

9

Availability and Accessibility

- The data collection protocol included two steps.

- First, world-wide-web, telephone directory, and city map searchers were conducted to identify city resources for physical activity participation
  - Schools
  - Parks
  - Fitness centers
  - Dance studios
  - Running paths

Availability and Accessibility

- Second, a number of agencies were contacted to provide global/geographic information system (GIS) data on physical activity resources and community characteristics.
  - County and City Parks and Recreation
  - The Metropolitan Planning Department
  - The City Police Department

Availability and Accessibility

- For the consistency of information gathered census tracts were used as the unit of analysis (n=37).
  - Census tracks that included both urban and rural areas were excluded (n=5)
  - Census tracks were matched based upon geographic area, population, and economic status
  - High and low SES areas were identified using a combination of employment rate, poverty rate, and average income within the tract

Availability and Accessibility

- **High SES (4 tracks, <u>n</u>=18,825)**
  - Per Capita Income= 21,126
  - 4.8 % below poverty level
  - 2.8% unemployment

- **Low SES (6 tracks, <u>n</u>=20,250)**
  - Per Capita Income= 8,582
  - 26.6 % below poverty level
  - 9.7% unemployment

Availability and Accessibility

Bar chart with categories Total, Pay, Free on the x-axis (scale 0–80) comparing High SES and Low SES.

Availability and Accessibility

- Areas with low and high SES did not differ in the amount of resources

- Accessibility…
  - 75% of resources are free of charge in high SES areas
  - 40% of the resources were pay facilities in low SES areas

- City planning appears to favor areas of high SES when providing physical activity resources such as free facilities, green space, and walkways

END

Chapter 12: Self Efficacy for Physical Activity

The Psychology of Physical Activity
Albert V. Carron
Heather A. Hausenblas
Paul A. Estabrooks

Confidence is a plant of slow growth
William Pitt

Self Efficacy

☼'Unless people believe they can produce
desired effects by their actions, they have
little incentive to act. Efficacy belief,
therefore, is a major basis for action'

☼Self-efficacy
➜ 'Beliefs in one's capabilities to organize and
execute courses of action required to produce
given attainments'

(Bandura, 1997)

Self Efficacy in Social Cognitive Theory

❀Social cognitive theory combines aspects of operant conditioning, social learning theory, and cognitive psychology

❀Triadic Reciprocal Causation

Self Efficacy in Social Cognitive Theory

❀Bandura's basic hypothesis of triadic reciprocation provides a framework for intervention development that targets both individual level cognitions and environmental variables as potential mediators of health behavior change.

Personal ←——→ Environmental

Behavior

Self Efficacy in Social Cognitive Theory

❀Implications of accepting a triadic reciprocal causation perspective
- ➡ Cognitions such as self-efficacy are assumed to play a role in behavior
- ➡ Learn through the consequences of own actions
- ➡ An individual's beliefs can be influenced by external environmental factors

Self Efficacy Sources and Outcomes

Clear success or failure performance experiences are the most powerful sources of self-efficacy information

Self Efficacy Sources and Outcomes

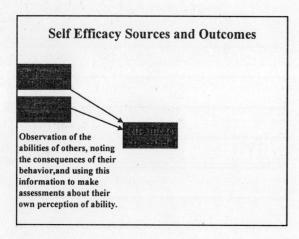

Observation of the abilities of others, noting the consequences of their behavior,and using this information to make assessments about their own perception of ability.

Self Efficacy Sources and Outcomes

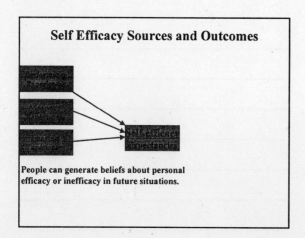

People can generate beliefs about personal efficacy or inefficacy in future situations.

Self Efficacy Sources and Outcomes

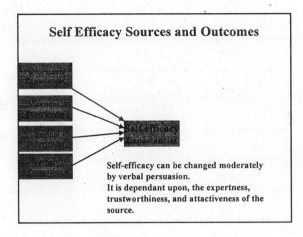

Self-efficacy can be changed moderately by verbal persuasion.
It is dependant upon, the expertness, trustworthiness, and attactiveness of the source.

Self Efficacy Sources and Outcomes

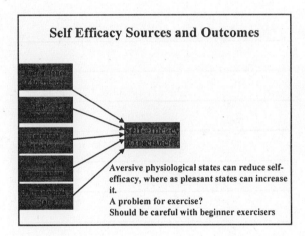

Aversive physiological states can reduce self-efficacy, where as pleasant states can increase it.
A problem for exercise?
Should be careful with beginner exercisers

Self Efficacy Sources and Outcomes

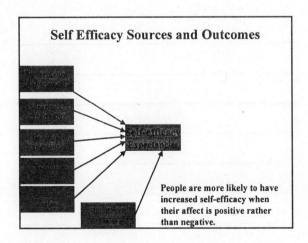

People are more likely to have increased self-efficacy when their affect is positive rather than negative.

Self Efficacy Sources and Outcomes

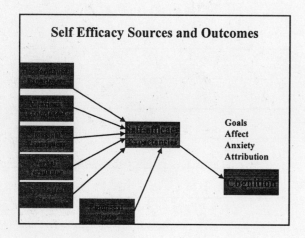

Goals
Affect
Anxiety
Attribution

Self Efficacy Sources and Outcomes

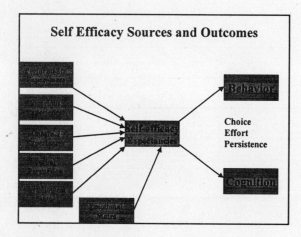

Choice
Effort
Persistence

Dimensions of Self-Efficacy

- Self-efficacy expectancies vary along three dimensions: magnitude, strength, and generality.
- Magnitude
  - The number of levels of increasing difficulty that a person believes himself to be capable of performing.

Dimensions of Self-Efficacy

Strength

➡ The firmness of one's convictions that he/she can perform the behavior in question

➡ For example two people may believe that they can attend an exercise class regularly, but one may have stronger convictions than the other

---

Dimensions of Self-Efficacy

Generality

➡ The generalizability of self-efficacy expectancies for a specific behavior to other behaviors within similar contexts

➡ For example a steel worker who does a lot of heavy lifting develops strong self-efficacy for his/her ability to lift heavy objects, could this generalize to his/her efficacy regarding weight lifting?

Self-Efficacy in Physical Activity Contexts

Edward McAuley and Shannon Mihalko (1998) identified four main categories:

➡ Exercise efficacy: beliefs about the capability of successfully engaging in incremental bouts of physical activity

➡ Barriers efficacy: beliefs about possessing the capability to overcome obstacles to physical activity

Self-Efficacy in Physical Activity Contexts

☼ Four main categories continued:

➡ Disease specific/health behavior efficacy: Similar to exercise efficacy but aimed at assessing efficacy beliefs in specific populations engaged in the secondary prevention of disease through exercise rehabilitation

➡ Perceived behavioral control: Beliefs about the degree of personal control in the decision to engage in physical activity

Initiation and Maintenance of Physical Activity

☼ Exercise efficacy=prediction of initiation

☼ Barrier efficacy= prediction of physical activity later in a program

☼ These findings hold with both younger and older adults

General Research Results

SE is related to:

☼ Choice of behavior

➡ Choice of exercise type
➡ Intention to exercise
➡ Initiation of exercise

☼ Effort exerted

➡ Ratings of perceived exertion
➡ Peak HR during exercise
➡ Self reports

☼ Adherence

➡ Long term maintenance
➡ Disease prevention programs

Self-efficacy And Mental States

🔔 **Higher perceptions of self-efficacy have been related to:**

➡ **Greater intention to be Physically Active**

➡ **Positive emotional responses**

➡ **More optimism**

➡ **Greater self-esteem**

END

Chapter 13: Health Belief Model, Protection Motivation Theory, and Physical Activity

The Psychology of Physical Activity
Albert V. Carron
Heather A. Hausenblas
Paul A. Estabrooks

Those who are enamored of practice without science are like a pilot who gets into a ship without a rudder or compass and never has any certainty of where he or she is going
Leonardo da Vinci

**Health Belief Model
(HBM)**

- One of the first models that adapted theory from the behavioral sciences to health problems

- Most widely recognized conceptual framework for health behavior

- Developed to encourage behaviors that prevent unwanted adverse conditions

Assumptions of the HBM

☼ For an individual to take action to avoid an unwanted health outcome, he she must feel …

➡ **Personally susceptible**
➡ **Disease will have at least moderate severity on some component of life**
➡ **By taking action, severity or susceptibility will be reduced**
➡ **Perceived benefits of doing the behavior will outweigh the perceived barriers**

Individual

Perceptions

perceived likelihood of contracting the disease

Perceived seriousness of disease in terms of contraction or non-treatment

---

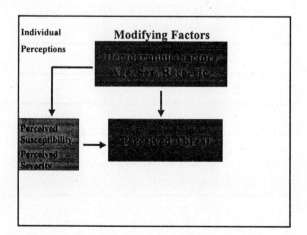

Individual   **Modifying Factors**

Perceptions

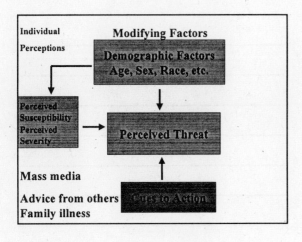

Individual Perceptions | Modifying Factors

Modifying Factors

Demographic Factors
Age, Sex, Race, etc.

Perceived Susceptibility
Perceived Severity

Perceived Threat

Mass media

Advice from others
Family illness

Cues to Action

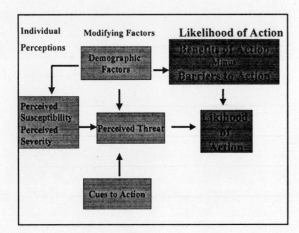

Individual Perceptions | Modifying Factors | **Likelihood of Action**

Demographic Factors

Benefits of Action Minus Barriers to Action

Perceived Susceptibility
Perceived Severity

Perceived Threat

Likihood of Action

Cues to Action

HBM and Physical Activity

Slecker and her colleagues (1984) examined the utility of the HBM for distinguishing joggers from non-exercisers

➡ Joggers= 3 times/wk for twenty minutes
➡ Non-exerciser= had not exercised regularly for the past six months
➡ Joggers=greater perception of severity, more benefits of and cues to jogging, and less barriers to jog
➡ Perceived susceptibility did not distinguish joggers and non-exercisers.

HBM and Physical Activity

- Desmond et al. (1990) assessed …
  - Exercise knowledge
  - Cues to action
  - Perceived severity of health risks
  - Perceived susceptibility to health risks
  - Benefits of exercise
  - Barriers to exercise

- 154 Black and 93 White fit and unfit adolescents.

HBM and Physical Activity

- Unfit (vs. fit) black students ….
  - Rated health problems from no exercise as more severe
- Unfit (vs. fit) white students ….
  - Rated susceptibility to health problems as greater
- Both contrary to health belief model

Is Health Belief Model Valid for Prediction of Exercise Behavior?

- Godin & Shephard (1990) carried out a narrative review

- Found no clear support for model in physical activity

- Why Not?

Limitations of the Health Belief Model...

- Reliance on health as the primary driving force behind exercise behavior.
- Developed to predict a single instance of a specific behavior acute (not chronic)
- Has not been applied in the appropriate manner
  - Primarily used as a behavior prediction model
  - A behavioral change model

Protection Motivation Theory

- Developed to explain inconsistencies in research on fear appeals and attitude change

- Concerned with the decision to protect oneself from harmful or stressful life events

- May also be viewed as a theory of coping

Protection Motivation Theory

- Decisions to engage (or not engage) in health-related behaviors based on:
  - Threat appraisal
  - Coping appraisal
  - Common index of protection motivation is a measure of intentions

Protection Motivation Theory

☼ Threat appraisal:

- ➡ An evaluation of the factors that influence the likelihood of engaging in a potentially unhealthy behavior
- ➡ Perceived vulnerability--estimate of the degree of personal risk for a specific health hazard if a current unhealthy behaviors is continued
- ➡ Perceived severity--estimate of the threat of the disease
- ➡ Continuation of unhealthy behavior is increased by the perceived intrinsic and extrinsic rewards of the unhealthy behavior

Protection Motivation Theory

☼ Coping appraisal:

- ➡ Response efficacy--expectancy that complying with recommendations will remove the threat
- ➡ Self-efficacy--belief in one's ability to implement the recommended coping behavior or strategy
- ➡ The likelihood of carrying out the preventive coping response is decreased by the perceived costs of completing the health behavior

Protection Motivation Theory Assumptions

☼ Motivation to implement the coping response is at its maximum when the individual perceives :

- ➡ The threat is severe
- ➡ He or she is personally vulnerable to the threat
- ➡ The coping response is effective to avert the threat
- ➡ He or she has the ability to perform the coping response

Protection Motivation Theory Research

- Meta-analysis carried out by Floyd and her colleagues (2000)

- 65 studies with 29,650 participants

- Adaptive intentions and behaviors were moderately facilitated by:
  - increases in threat severity
  - threat vulnerability
  - response efficacy
  - self-efficacy

Protection Motivation and Physical Activity

- Plotnikoff and Higginbotham (1998) examined the prediction of diet and physical activity to prevent further cardiovascular heart disease in 151 recent heart attack patients
  - Completed baseline measures of threat appraisal following a heart attack
  - Six months later completed measures of threat appraisal and coping appraisal
  - Self-efficacy was the strongest predictor of exercise and diet intentions and behaviors
  - Concluded that health education for this population should promote self-efficacy enhancing activities for such behaviors

---

Protection Motivation and Physical Activity

- Courneya (1995) compared perceptions of the severity of a sedentary lifestyle among 270 senior citizens who were classified within one of the five stages of the Transtheoretical Model.
  - Precontemplation
  - Contemplation
  - Preparation
  - Action
  - Maintenance

Protection Motivation and Physical Activity

※ Found:

➡ Precontemplation stage reported the least perceived severity of the consequences of an inactive lifestyle

※ Concluded that the main function of perceived severity of physical inactivity is to motivate people to seriously consider becoming physically active

END

Chapter 14: The Theories of Reasoned Action and Planned Behavior and Physical Activity

The Psychology of Physical Activity
Albert V. Carron
Heather A. Hausenblas
Paul A. Estabrooks

Man can alter his life by altering his thinking
William James

Two Theories

- Two social-cognitive theories have guided the majority of theory-based research on physical activity
  - Theory of Reasoned Action
  - Theory of Planned Behavior

- Both:
  - Reflect an expectation by value approach
  - Assume individuals are capable of forethought and make rational decisions

Theory of Reasoned Action
Fishbein & Ajzen (1975)

- Applicable to volitional behaviors
- Assumes that people:
  - make systematic use of the information available to them
  - consider the implications of the behavior before engaging in behavior

---

Theory of Reasoned Action

- Three principal constructs considered to influence behavior:
  - Intention
  - Attitude
  - Subjective norm
- Intention
  - Direct determinant of behavior
  - What an individual plans to do
  - Remain stable over a short period
  - Product of attitude and subjective norm

Theory of Reasoned Action

- Attitude:
  - positive or negative evaluation of performing the behavior
  - behavioral beliefs
    - Expected outcome: belief that exercise will lead or will not lead to a given outcome
    - Outcome value: positive or negative evaluation placed on the outcome

Theory of Reasoned Action

☼ **Subjective Norm:**

➡ Person's perceived pressures from individuals or groups to perform or not perform the behavior

➡ normative beliefs

➢ Strength component: perceptions of expectations of important others

➢ Motivation to comply: with those expectations

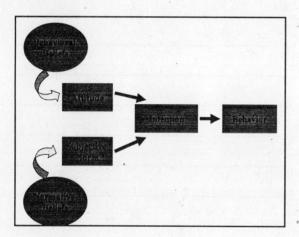

Limitations of Theory of Reasoned Action

☼ Not appropriate for predicting or explaining behavior in situations where people had little power over events around them

☼ If a behavior is not fully under volition control a person may be highly motivated by high attitudes and subjective norm yet may not perform the behavior

Theory of Planned Behavior

- To improve the predictive power of the Theory of Reasoned Action Ajzen added a third construct to the original theory

- Perceived behavioral control

- This reflects the fundamental difference between the theory of reasoned action and the theory of planned behavior

---

Theory of Planned Behavior
Ajzen (1985)

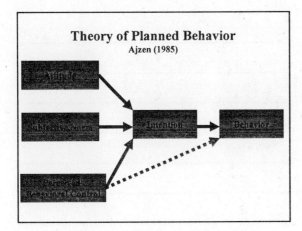

Perceived Behavioral Control

- Perceived ease or difficulty in performing a behavior

- Extent that non-volitional factors interfere with ones' attempt to perform a behavior

- Made up of control beliefs
  - facilitating and obstructing factors
  - perceived power of a control factor to facilitate or inhibit the behavior

Elicitation Studies

☼ **Determine the pertinent beliefs concerning a behavior by:**
  ➡ Using open-ended questions to assess behavioral, normative, and control beliefs in the targeted population
  ➡ Carrying out a content analysis to identify which beliefs are most salient
  ➡ Developing structured items from the content analysis
  ➡ Making items specific to the target, action, context, and time

Elicitation Studies

☼ **Courneya and Friedenreich (1999) the salient beliefs of 24 breast cancer survivors:**
  ➡ Women answered open-ended questions about exercising during their cancer treatment
  ➡ Listed the main advantages and disadvantages
  ➡ Listed factors that prevented or helped them
  ➡ Listed individuals or groups who were most important to them when they thought about exercising during treatment

Elicitation Studies

☼ **Found salient behavioral beliefs were:**
  ➡ Gets my mind off cancer and treatment
  ➡ Makes me feel better and improves my well-being
  ➡ Helps me maintain a normal lifestyle
  ➡ Helps me cope with my life and the stress over cancer
  ➡ Helps in my recovery from surgery and treatment
  ➡ Helps me control my weight

Elicitation Studies

☼ Found salient sources for normative beliefs were:
- ➡ Spouse
- ➡ Other family members
- ➡ Friends
- ➡ Physicians
- ➡ Other persons with cancer

Elicitation Studies

☼ Found salient control beliefs were:
- ➡ Nausea experienced
- ➡ Fatigue/tiredness experienced
- ➡ Lack of time to exercise
- ➡ Lack of support for exercise
- ➡ Pain and soreness experienced
- ➡ Lack of counseling for exercise
- ➡ Work at regular job

☼ In sum the procedure revealed that the salient beliefs of breast cancer patients concerning exercise were different from those of healthy populations

Theories of Reasoned Action and Planned Behavior
Meta-Analysis

☼ Hausenblas, Carron, & Mack (1997)

☼ 31 studies

☼ Recall effect sizes (ES)
- ➡ Small ES = .20
- ➡ Moderate ES = .50
- ➡ Large ES = .80

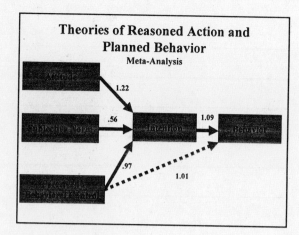

Theories of Reasoned Action and Planned Behavior
Meta-Analysis

Potential Limitations of the Theories

- Factors such as personality and demographic variables are not directly considered
- Ambiguity regarding how to define and measure perceived behavioral control
- Long time intervals between intention and behavior reduce the chance of prediction
- The utility of subjective norm is questionable

END

Chapter 15: The Transtheoretical Model and Physical Activity

The Psychology of Physical Activity
Albert V. Carron
Heather A. Hausenblas
Paul A. Estabrooks

One size does not fit all

Transtheoretical Model (TTM)

- Changing unhealthy behaviors is challenging

- Change is lengthy process, involves progressing through several stages

- "One size <u>does not</u> fit all" philosophy forms basis of TTM

- Integrative model of of behavior change born out of the combination of over 300 theories of psychotherapy

- TTM comprised of 5 constructs

TTM

🔔 **Five constructs of the TTM include:**

1. Stages of Change
2. Decisional Balance
3. Processes of Change in TTM
4. Self-efficacy
5. Temptation

Stages of Change

🔔 **Major contribution of TTM to health field is behavior change takes time through a series of stages**

🔔 **Three aspects:**
- ➡ Stages fall somewhere between traits & states
- ➡ Stages are both stable & dynamic in nature
- ➡ There are six stages which people pass through in attempting any health behavior change

Stages of Change Model

Behavior change involves moving through six stages

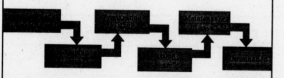

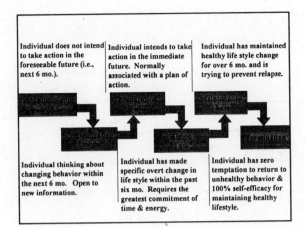

Individual does not intend to take action in the foreseeable future (i.e., next 6 mo.).

Individual intends to take action in the immediate future. Normally associated with a plan of action.

Individual has maintained healthy life style change for over 6 mo. and is trying to prevent relapse.

Individual thinking about changing behavior within the next 6 mo. Open to new information.

Individual has made specific overt change in life style within the past six mo. Requires the greatest commitment of time & energy.

Individual has zero temptation to return to unhealthy behavior & 100% self-efficacy for maintaining healthy lifestyle.

Decisional Balance

☼ "Balance sheet" assesses the importance an individual places on <u>pros</u> or <u>cons</u> of a behavior

☼ Balance between pros & cons varies depending on stage

☼ When cons are of greater importance than pro's, motivation to change behavior is low

---

Decisional Balance Across Stages

Pros < Cons   Pros = Cons   Pros > Cons

Pros < Cons   Pros > Cons

Processes of Change in TTM

🔔 Represents behaviors, cognitions, & emotions people engage in during course of changing behavior

🔔 Ten processes of change have received the most empirical support (Prochaska & Velicer, 1997)

_____

_____

_____

_____

_____

_____

_____

Processes of Change in TTM

1) **Gathering Information:** determining pros & cons of + behavior
2) **Making substitutions:** sedentary behavior with activity
3) **Being moved emotionally:** experiencing & expressing feelings about consequences of being active
4) **Being a role model:** considering how inactivity affects significant others
5) **Getting social support:** getting support for your intention to exercise

_____

_____

_____

_____

_____

_____

Processes of Change in TTM

6) **Developing a healthy self-image:** appraising one's self-image as a healthy regular exerciser
7) **Taking advantage of social mores:** social policy, customs
8) **Being rewarded:** reward oneself or rewarded by others for making changes
9) **Using cues:** using cues to engage in physical activity
10) **Making a commitment:** being committed to regular exercise

_____

_____

_____

_____

_____

_____

Processes of Change in Use

Television spot in California--

A middle aged man, clearly in distress says....

"I always worried that my smoking would lead to lung cancer. I was always afraid that my smoking would lead to an early death. But I never imagined that it would happen to my wife."

Then on the screen the following message is shown...

50,000 deaths per year are due to passive smoking.

Processes of Change in Use

- Gathering Information--50,000 deaths per year
- Being Moved Emotionally-- around grief, guilt, and fear that can be reduced if appropriate action is taken
- Developing a healthy self-image-- how do I think and feel about myself as a smoker
- Being a role model-- how do I feel and think about the effects of my smoking on my environment

---

Self-Efficacy

- Judgment regarding one's ability to perform behavior required to achieve a certain outcome
  - Proposed to change with each stage
  - Gorely & Gordon (1995) found barrier self-efficacy increased from precontemplation to contemplation to preparation to action to maintenance
  - Sullum et al. (2000) found students who become inactive over an 8 weeks had lower self-efficacy at baseline than those who maintained exercise level

Temptation

☼ **Represents intensity of the urges to engage in a specific behavior when in midst of difficult situations** (Grimley et al., 1994)

☼ **Research examining temptation in physical activity is limited**

☼ **Hausenblas et al. (in review) found a negative relationship between temptations to not exercise & self-efficacy**

☼ **They found maintainers had lowest temptation to not exercise & highest confidence in engaging in exercise**

Advantages of TTM

☼ **Three advantages of dividing population into stages of change:**

➡ **Provides opportunity to match intervention to needs of individuals in each stage**
➡ **Provides opportunity to subdivide at-risk population into precontemplation, contemplation, & preparation stages**
➡ **Recruitment & retention**

Research Support for TTM

☼ **Culos-Reed et al. (2001) noted research using TTM can be classified into 3 categories:**
➡ **Studies combining stages of change w/ other social-cognitive models**
➡ **Cross-sectional studies examining various TTM constructs**
➡ **Intervention studies**

Stages of Change & Social Cognitive Models

※ Courneya (1995) examined the relationship between perceived severity & stages of change

※ Found perceived severity of the consequences of an inactive lifestyle were less for individuals in the precontemplation stage than those in the contemplation stage

Cross-Sectional Studies

※ Nigg & Courneya (1998) studied 819 high school students & their stage of change.

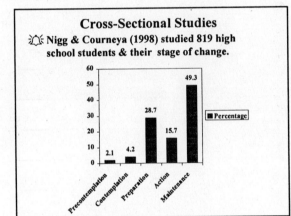

Intervention Research

※ Marcus et al. (1998) used TTM to increase initiation, adoption, & maintenance of physical activity of 1,559 employees

※ Employee randomly assigned to a stage-matched or standard self-help group

※ After 3 months those in stage-matched group had more positive changes

※ More individuals in self-help group failed to progress to another stage or even showed regression to an earlier stage

7

END

Chapter 16: Motivational Theories and Physical Activity

The Psychology of Physical Activity
Albert V. Carron
Heather A. Hausenblas
Paul A. Estabrooks

I know not the course others may take:
but as for me, give me liberty or give
me death.
Patrick Henry

Motivation

- Derived from the Latin word movere

- "to move"

- Psychological construct used to account for the why of behavior

- The selection of specific activities over others reflects underlying motivation

- Self-determination and Personal investment represent two theories of motivation

Self-Determination Theory

- ☼ Origins in the study of intrinsic vs. extrinsic motivation
- ☼ The impact of rewards on motivation
- ☼ Rewards can be perceived in two ways:
  - ➡ Information about competence
  - ➡ Information about control

Rewards as Control: An Illustration

- ☼ Children began playing baseball and making a great deal of noise in a neighborhood.
- ☼ An old man hated the noise and thought of a plan— he offered each child 25 cents if they would return and play.
- ☼ Children returned, played, and were paid.
- ☼ After paying for a few days the old man said it was too expensive and offered only 15¢
- ☼ After a few days, he asked them to continue for 5¢
- ☼ They refused and said they wouldn't play for 5¢

Sources of Motivation

NO MOTIVATION

EXTRINSIC MOTIVATION

INTRINSIC MOTIVATION

Sources of Motivation

☼Extrinsic motives

➡ **External regulation:** Person does activity to avoid punishment or receive reward

➡ **Introjeted regulation:** Partial internalization of behavior person does because he/she should or must

➡ **Identified regulation:** Person freely chooses activity not because of enjoyment but because it's important to do so

---

Sources of Motivation

☼Intrinsic motives

➡ **To learn:** To learn something new about the activity or the self

➡ **Accomplish tasks:** To obtain a sense of accomplishment

➡ **Experience Sensations:** To experience the pleasant sensations of the activity

---

Antecedents of Motivation

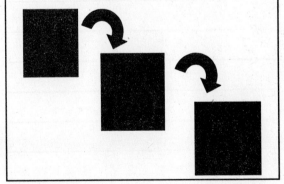

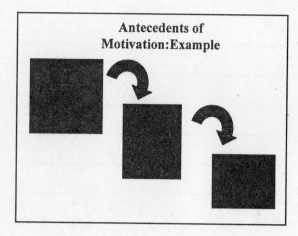

Antecedents of
Motivation:Example

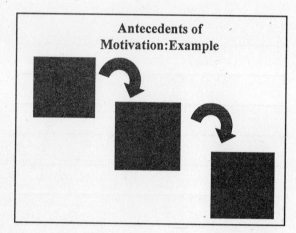

Antecedents of
Motivation:Example

Self-determination Theory
(Deci & Ryan, 1991)

- Self-determination theory hypothesizes that psychological mediators function between individual motives and motivation

- Psychological mediators reflect 3 psychological needs:
  - Autonomy -- control of our own actions
  - Competence -- be effective in our environment
  - Relatedness -- to feel connected to others

Self-Determination and Physical Activity

- Li (1999) tested 371 males and females who varied in frequency of exercise behavior

- Females report higher intrinsic motivation compared to males

- Higher frequency of physical activity was positively related to higher levels of intrinsic motivation

---

Self-Determination and Physical Activity

- Chatzisarantis & Biddle (1998) assessed two groups of adults

  → Controlling group -- external regulation (bad health) and introjected regulation (worry about health) motives

  → Autonomy group -- accomplishment (do well in PA) and experience stimulation (fun) motives

---

Self-Determination and Physical Activity

- Chatzisarantis & Biddle found that the autonomy group:

  → Were more involved in physical activity
  → Enjoyed physical activity more
  → Had more positive attitudes about physical activity
  → Perceived they had more personal control over physical activity

Self-Determination and Physical Activity

☼ Mullen & Markland (1997) examined if individuals at different stages of change differed in perceptions of self-determination

- ➡ Tested adults in mid 30s and categorized them into 5 stages of change on basis of physical activity patterns
- ➡ Also assessed motives for physical activity

Self-Determination and Physical Activity

☼ Mullen & Markland (1997) found that:

- ➡ Individuals in Precontemplation, Contemplation, Preparation Perceived themselves to be less self determined than individuals in Action and Maintenance
- ➡ Individuals in Precontemplation, Contemplation, Preparation had more 'ought to' & 'must do' motives.
- ➡ Individuals in Action and Maintenance had more 'Enjoy' & 'Like' motives

Personal Investment Theory
Maehr (1984)

☼ Developed to understand and promote school achievement

☼ Cognitive motivational theory

☼ Takes into account both the situation and the individual as determinants of behavior

☼ Attempts to integrate numerous achievement motivation propositions and models

Personal Investment Theory

- Amount of personal investment in a situation influences amount of personal resources used

- Motivation differs according to an individual's personal meaning associated with the situation

---

Assumptions of Personal Investment Theory

- The study of motivation is the study of behavior
- Individual patterns of behavior reflect personal investment
- Personal investment is reflected in choice of behavior
- Personal investment determined by meaning in a situation.
- This meaning and its origins can be determined and assessed

---

Factors Influencing a Situation's Meaning

- Sense of self -- an individual's collection of thoughts, beliefs, and feelings about who he or she is

- Perceived options – the behavioral alternatives believed to be available

- Personal incentives – the motivational focus of the activity

Personal Investment Theory

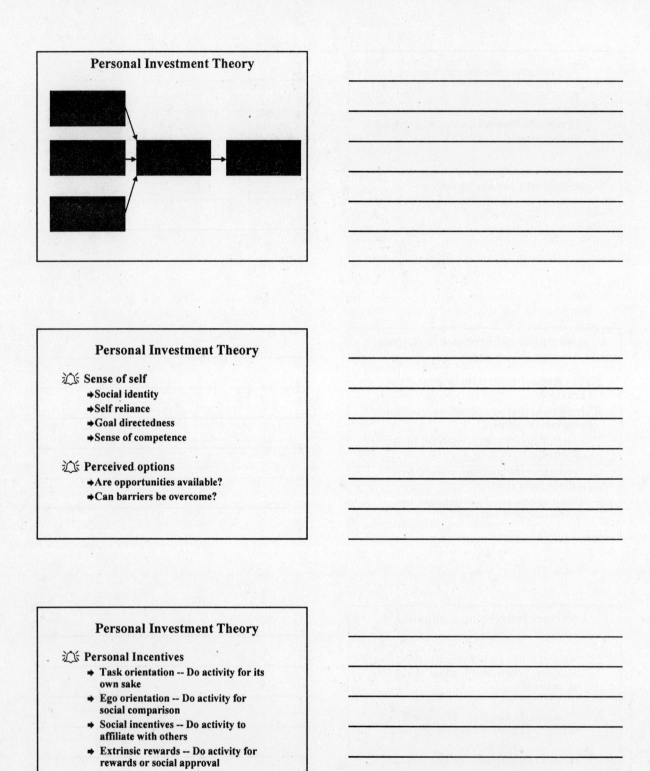

Personal Investment Theory

☼ **Sense of self**
  ➜ Social identity
  ➜ Self reliance
  ➜ Goal directedness
  ➜ Sense of competence

☼ **Perceived options**
  ➜ Are opportunities available?
  ➜ Can barriers be overcome?

Personal Investment Theory

☼ **Personal Incentives**
  ➜ Task orientation -- Do activity for its own sake
  ➜ Ego orientation -- Do activity for social comparison
  ➜ Social incentives -- Do activity to affiliate with others
  ➜ Extrinsic rewards -- Do activity for rewards or social approval

Personal Investment Theory and Physical Activity

🔔 Duda et al. (1989) measured attendance, completion of exercise protocols , and exercise intensity of injured intercollegiate athletes (n=40).

🔔 Found that Increased attendance was associated with increased personal incentives (social support, task involvement) and a better sense of self (self-motivation)

Personal Investment Theory and Physical Activity

🔔 Tappe et al. (1990) investigated the utility of personal investment theory to predict current level of physical activity in 237 adolescents

🔔 Found that males self identity and perceived options significant predictors of current activity

---

END

Chapter 17: Individual Level Intervention Strategies

The Psychology of Physical Activity
Albert V. Carron
Heather A. Hausenblas
Paul A. Estabrooks

If the human mind was simple enough to understand we'd be too simple to understand it.
Emerson Pugh

Individual Level Interventions

※ The study of behavior change in individuals is a core area of psychology

※ Behavior change interventions focusing on increasing or maintaining regular physical activity reflect the developmental ideas of psychology

Individual Level Interventions

- Early psychopathologists felt that behavioral anomalies reflected the external manifestation of evil spirits that had entered the victim's body

- A physical inactivity demon?

- "Hello, Mr. Jones, I think a ½ inch bit should do the trick"

- Luckily, behavior change interventions have advanced considerably

Interventions Defined

- Health-promoting activities that originate from a health promotion team with the intention of instilling or maintaining health-related attitudes, norms, and behaviors, in a specific target (Gauvin, Levesque, & Richard, 2001)

Interventions Defined

- Efficacy trials provide "a test of whether a technology, treatment, procedure, or program does more good than harm when delivered under optimum conditions"

- For example, randomly assigning sedentary individuals to either an exercise intervention or no-exercise control group

Interventions Defined

- Effectiveness trials are "tests of whether a technology, treatment, procedure, intervention, or program does more good than harm when delivered under real-world conditions"

- For example, a physical activity intervention that was shown to be efficacious is tested in a community with volunteer leaders

_____

_____

_____

_____

_____

_____

Individual Interventions for Physical Activity

- Dishman and Buckworth (1996) located 127 studies that had approximately 131,000 subjects who had been targeted in community, worksite, school, home, and health care settings

- Studies tested interventions designed to increase physical activity

_____

_____

_____

_____

_____

_____

Individual Interventions for Physical Activity

- The authors expressed the effect sizes as Pearson correlation coefficients (r).

- Correlation values of .10, .30, and .50 are considered small, medium, and large effects, respectively.

_____

_____

_____

_____

_____

_____

Individual Interventions for Physical Activity

Effect size

r= 0	r=.20	r=.40	r=.60	r = .80

→

50%	60%	70%	80%	100%

% chance of intervention adherence

Individual Interventions for Physical Activity

🔔 Beneficial impact of an intervention program was identical for:
- ➡ Males and females
- ➡ Individuals of different ages
- ➡ Whites and nonwhites (i.e., African Americans, Mexican Americans, and Native Americans)

Individual Interventions for Physical Activity

🔔 The effect of interventions differed for healthy participants when contrasted with all groups of patients

🔔 An important qualifier: only a relatively small number of studies examined interventions with patients.

Individual Interventions for Physical Activity

☼ **Dishman and Buckworth noted that there were several types of interventions that have been used**

☼ **Completed comparisons between 7 general categories of interventions.**

Types of Individual Interventions

☼ **Behavior modification**
  ➡ Interventions that manipulate antecedent conditions and consequences of performing or not performing a behavior
☼ **Cognitive Behavior modification**
  ➡ Interventions that include self-monitoring, self-reinforcement, cognitive restructuring
☼ **Health education**
  ➡ Individual given information about risks and benefits of physical activity

---

Types of Individual Interventions

☼ **Health-risk appraisal**
  ➡ individual confronted with results from health risk appraisal
☼ **Exercise prescription**
  ➡ individual given exercise programs of moderate intensity
☼ **Physical education curriculum**
  ➡ education programs implemented in the school system
☼ **Combinations of programs that include two or more distinct interventions**

Type of Intervention and Physical Activity

- Behavior modification (r=.91)
- Cognitive behavior modification (r=.10)
- Health education/risk appraisal (r=.10)
- Exercise prescription (r=.21)
- Physical education curriculum (r=.21)
- Combinations (r=.11)

Behavior Modification

- Operant conditioning techniques attributed to B. F. Skinner (1947)

- Conditions are called antecedents in that they come before a behavior occurs
  → For example a stop sign=a cue to stop

- Once cued by an antecedent it is thought that a behavior or response will occur
  → See stop sign then stop

Behavior Modification

- The final component of operant conditioning is the consequence of the response

- Scenario 1: A driver approaches a stop sign at a new intersection. It is the driver's first experience with this stop sign and so he/she stops. The driver notices a heavy flow of traffic on the intersecting street. This acts as the reinforcing consequence that will ensure the driver will stop next time he/she encounters this stop sign

6

Behavior Modification

Scenario 2: A driver approaches a stop sign on a quiet corner of his neighborhood. The driver has seen this stop sign many times before and has never seen traffic on the intersecting street. In this scenario, there is no reinforcing consequence associated with coming to a complete stop (assuming there are no police close by!) but there is a reinforcing consequence to not stopping (saved time). It is likely that the antecedent cue of this stop sign is not enough to elicit the stopping behavior in this scenario

Behavior Modification

Roger Katz and Nirbhay Singh (1986) used both stimulus control and reinforcement to increase recess physical activity of handicapped children

Stimulus control=a large colorful poster was placed in a high profile area of the playground during the two recess periods

The poster showed images of Freddy and Freena Frog playing ball games and climbing on the jungle gym

Behavior Modification

Reinforcement
  ➡ Verbal praise for being physically active

  ➡ Active children became members of the Freddy and Freena club

  ➡ Photographs were taken daily and four pictures of active children on the playground were placed on the large poster

Approach to Delivery of Interventions

- Face-to-face programs -- delivered directly to the individual

- Mediated approach -- delivered indirectly by mail or telephone

- Mediated approaches produce better results

Setting of Interventions

- When compared to home, school, or health-care setting interventions general community based interventions produce better results

- Interventions delivered in the presence of others are superior than those delivered to people on their own

- Unsupervised interventions produce better results than supervised interventions

Type of Physical Activity Targeted

- Interventions that promote leisure time physical activity are more successful than those that promote strength or aerobic exercise

- Interventions that promote moderate intensity physical activity are more successful than those that promote strenuous activities

Interventions Based On Theoretical Models

- Baranowski and his associates (1998) located 25 studies that had employed at least one theory as the guiding framework for the intervention

- Concluded that interventions based on a theory are superior to a-theoretical interventions

- Unfortunately, the interventions is sum have a small effect on physical activity

Interventions Based On Theoretical Models

- Baranowski et al. (1998) suggested that:
  - interventions work by means of mediating variable
  - current theoretical models from which mediating variables are obtained often do not account for substantial variability in the target outcomes
  - interventions have not been shown to effect substantial change in the mediating variables
  - these factors impose limits on the effectiveness of interventions

Interventions Based On Theoretical Models

- Baranowski et al. (1998) suggested two priorities for physical activity intervention research:

  - It is necessary to fully understand the relationships between theoretical mediators and physical activity
  - The impact of interventions on these mediating variables should be examined

Individual Level Interventions And Technological Advances

- ☼ Strategic planning of individual level interventions using technological advances increases the ability to individualize interventions on a large scale and the number of channels available for program delivery

- ☼ Expert systems are a good example of such an advance

END

Chapter 18: Group Level Intervention Strategies

The Psychology of Physical Activity
Albert V. Carron
Heather A. Hausenblas
Paul A. Estabrooks

Coming together is a beginning, staying together is progress, working together is success.
Henry Ford

Group Level Intervention Strategies

- People do come together and engage in physical activity programs in group settings in private fitness clubs, community centers, universities, and so on.

- Some maintain their involvement

- But, what about working together— what Ford called success?

1

Group Level Intervention Strategies

🔔 Zander (1982) suggested that a collection of individuals can be classified as a group when they:
  ➡ Converse freely
  ➡ Identify the collective as "we" and other collectives as "they"
  ➡ Attend and actively participate in group functions
  ➡ Are primarily interested in group, not personal accomplishments
  ➡ Are interested in the progress of the collective

The Dyersville Experience

🔔 The Beginning

  ➡ The first step in the project was to bring people together.
  ➡ Advertised a program for community members interested in losing weight within a supportive social environment.
  ➡ Over 450 participants in a town of 3,800!

🔔 Ford's beginning had been realized—participants had come together.

The Dyersville Experience

🔔 The Progress

  ➡ Strategies to assist the participants in their efforts to maintain involvement in the weekly diet, physical activity, and motivational sessions
  ➡ Participants were assigned to teams
  ➡ Teams decided a name and T-shirts
  ➡ Participants enjoyed the weekly meetings and were rarely absent

🔔 Progress also had been realized—participants stayed together

The Dyersville Experience

- THE SUCCESS!!
- Based on weight loss
- Entire teams stepped onto a giant truck scale to monitor their progress
- The winning teams were those that had lost the most collective weight.
- How successful was the Dyersville campaign?
- The 450 plus participants lost a combined 7,500 pounds!

_____

_____

_____

_____

_____

_____

_____

Theoretical Foundation for Group Level Physical Activity Interventions

- The Dyersville project was not a scientific study
- Why did the project work?
- What were the group processes that facilitated behavior change?
- What components were necessary to ensure sustained participation?
- Will such a program ensure long-term adherence to healthy eating and/or physical activity?

_____

_____

_____

_____

_____

_____

Theoretical Foundation for Group Level Physical Activity Interventions

- Carron and Spink (1993) proposed a conceptual framework for the application of group dynamics' principles in physical activity classes

- Based on the assumption that various inputs and throughputs can lead to desired outputs in group settings

- Based upon the tenet that adherence is associated with perceptions of cohesiveness

_____

_____

_____

_____

_____

_____

Theoretical Foundation for Group Level Physical Activity Interventions

- The inputs = the group environment and structure
  - Distinctiveness
  - Class norms
  - Geographical position

- The throughputs = group processes
  - Interaction
  - Communications
  - Sacrifices by members for the collective

- The output = increased perceptions of cohesion

Theoretical Foundation for Group Level Physical Activity Interventions

- In Dyersville
  - Weight-loss teams also were encouraged to select a catchy name and have t-shirts made = feelings of distinctiveness
  - Members developed common expectations around collective goals = group norms
  - The length of the program provided ample time for the development of group interaction and communication = group processes

Team Building in Physical Activity Settings

- Carron and Spink (1993) first applied their framework to female participants in 17 university aerobic fitness classes

- Classes met 3 times/week for 13 weeks

- Randomly assigned to either a team-building or control condition

- A four-stage process consisting of an introductory, a conceptual, a practical, and an intervention stage

Team Building in Physical Activity Settings

- Introductory stage--20-minute presentation to class instructors

- Conceptual stage--provided the class instructors with an understanding of the conceptual framework

- Practical stage--the class instructors become active agents in the development of specific strategies

- Intervention stage--specific intervention strategies were introduced and maintained throughout the program

---

Team Building in Physical Activity Settings

- The intervention was successful: team-building increased perceptions of cohesion

- Individuals in the team-building and control conditions did not differ on attendance

- Fewer drop outs from classes that had experienced the team-building intervention and participants were less likely to be late

---

Team Building in Physical Activity Settings

- How do these findings generalize?

- Previous research has shown that exercise class cohesion can be improved through team-building techniques

- As cohesion is a predictor of exercise participation in older exercisers, a similar intervention should improve adherence to an exercise class developed for older adults

Team Building in Physical Activity Settings

☀ **Estabrooks & Carron (1999) examined the effect of a team-building intervention on exercise attendance and program return rate of older adult exercisers**

☀ **Participants were first time registrants in a fitness program for seniors.**

☀ **Physical activity classes met for 1 hour 2 times per week for 6 weeks.**

Team Building in Physical Activity Settings

☀ **Participants were randomly assigned to the team-building, attention-placebo, or control condition.**

☀ **The control condition received a standard-care physical activity class.**

☀ **The attention-placebo condition received a standard-care physical activity class plus a weekly visit from a research assistant.**

Team Building in Physical Activity Settings

☀ **The team-building intervention was based upon strategies from group dynamics:**

➡ **Promote distinctiveness**
➡ **Introduce roles within the group**
➡ **Set group goals**
➡ **Foster increased interaction and communication among group members**

Carron & Spink, 1993

Team Building in Physical Activity Settings

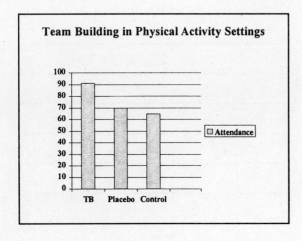

Team Building in Physical Activity Settings

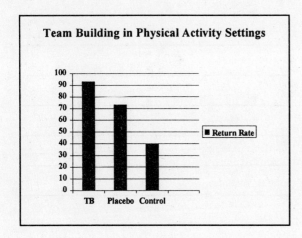

Team Building in Physical Activity Settings

- Annesi (1999) -- changes in participation rates might be the result of leader attention

- Examined the effectiveness of a group cohesion based intervention when there is minimal leader contact

- New members of the facility participated

- All given the standard orientation and prescribed a 3-time weekly exercise program lasting 15 weeks

Team Building in Physical Activity Settings

- ☼ The participants in the intervention arm attended more sessions (65% vs 48%) and had less drop-out (29% vs 50%)

- ☼ It was concluded that simply having new exercisers warm-up and cool down together should increase the probability of program adherence

---

Concerns About Group-based Interventions

- ☼ King and her associates (1998) questioned utility of group-based approaches

- ☼ May be effective for short-term but counter productive for long-term participation
  - ➡ Participants could become dependent upon the group environment for sustained participation
  - ➡ Programs invariably end either for a summer or winter break or because the program's objectives have been met
  - ➡ Those individuals who depend upon the group's support may cease to be physically active if/when the group ceases to exist

---

Concerns About Group-based Interventions

- ☼ Does the above concern have merit?
  - ➡ Studies rarely, if ever, report physical activity rates once the program ends
  - ➡ Estabrooks and Carron (1999) did not assess physical activity between the completion of the 1st program and the initiation of the 2nd
  - ➡ Participants may have become relatively or completely inactive during the hiatus
  - ➡ The participants might not have the confidence or skills necessary to complete a similar program at home

Concerns About Group-based Interventions

🔔 The question that remains is—can group-based intervention continue to exert an influence on independent individual behavior after the group ceases to exist?

Group-Based Interventions as Agents of Change

🔔 Brawley and his associates (2000) examined if a group-based intervention could be effective for increasing individual participation not only during the life of the program but also when the program was terminated

🔔 Healthy previously sedentary older adults (> 65 years) were recruited and assigned to one of three conditions— group-motivated cognitive-behavioral, standard physical activity, or wait-list control

---

Group-Based Interventions as Agents of Change

🔔 The study was carried out in three periods of 3 months each

🔔 Throughout those periods questionnaires were administered to assess levels of physical activity and perceptions about quality of life

Group-Based Interventions as Agents of Change

☼ 1st 3-month period, the intervention was introduced

☼ The group-motivated cognitive-behavioral condition and the standard physical activity condition participated in a structured program that included physical activities at home

☼ Individuals in these two conditions were exposed to considerably different sets of experiences

Group-Based Interventions as Agents of Change

☼ The intervention used with the group-motivated cognitive-behavioral condition included many components of Carron and Spink's (1993) conceptual model

Group-Based Interventions as Agents of Change

☼ The participants selected and adopted a group name

☼ Told that their group was "above average" in their members' potential to change

☼ Facilitated interaction and communication

☼ Taught a number of self-regulatory skills and then asked to pair up for the purpose of practicing the new skills

☼ Group relevant goals for monitoring and behavior

Group-Based Interventions as Agents of Change

- The group discussed individual and group goals, possible reasons for failure associated with the

- The participants were also encouraged to begin discussing how to maintain individual physical activity

- The group discussed the implications of decreasing contact between the project staff and participants.

_____

_____

_____

_____

_____

_____

_____

Group-Based Interventions as Agents of Change

- In the final 3-month period, the program was terminated

- The participants in the group-mediated cognitive-behavioral condition
  - Higher average frequency of physical activity
  - Greater total amount of physical activity during the initial 6 months of the intervention
  - Maintained a higher rate of activity 9 months after the completion of the program

_____

_____

_____

_____

_____

_____

_____

END

_____

_____

_____

_____

_____

_____

_____

Chapter 19: Community Level Intervention Strategies

The Psychology of Physical Activity
Albert V. Carron
Heather A. Hausenblas
Paul A. Estabrooks

In communities where men build ships for their own sons to fish or fight from, quality is never a problem.
J. A. Dever

Community Level Interventions

❧ Community strategies typically include a number of institutions, organizations, and groups to deliver a variety of interventions

❧ Target system change rather than individual behavior change

Community Level Interventions

☼ Karen Glanz (1997) provided an outline of the benefit and breadth of community level interventions

- ➡ Community-level models suggest strategies and initiatives that are panned and led by organizations and institutions whose missions are to protect and improve health: schools, worksites, health care settings, community groups, and governmental agencies. Other institutions for whom health enhancement is not a central mission, such as the mass media, also play a critical role.

Community Defined

☼ An aggregate of people who share common values and institutions

☼ Shared institutions include: local hospitals, recreation centers, worksites, faith-based institutions, and schools

☼ Refers to the locality of an aggregate of people, groups or institutions

☼ Informal social norms, belief systems, interdependent groups, and attachments

Why Focus on Communities?

☼ There is practicality in developing and implementing physical activity interventions at the community level

- ➡ A community-based intervention should increase level of quality and time invested into health promotion because of the inter-group relationships, shared values, and a common attachment within the community

Community Interventions

◆ Community programs for the promotion of physical activity

◆ 4 primary sections:
  ➡ Site-based interventions
  ➡ Community-wide and policy interventions
  ➡ Mass media interventions
  ➡ The Centers for Disease Control and Prevention guidelines for community-based physical activity interventions.

Site-Based Interventions: Schools

◆ Elementary, middle, and high schools have traditionally offered physical education classes

◆ Schools are offering fewer, and shorter duration, physical education classes and have even eliminated them completely is some cases

---

Site-Based Interventions: Schools

◆ Two Areas of Focus:
  ◆ Increasing physical activity during physical education classes
  ◆ Increasing out-of-school physical activity

◆ Stone and associates (1998) examined the effectiveness of 14 school interventions

Site-Based Interventions: Schools

❁Stone and associates found:
  ➡ **Interventions were often successful at improving knowledge and attitudes towards physical activity**
  ➡ **Interventions were typically successful at increasing physical activity during physical education classes**
  ➡ **Interventions were often unsuccessful at increasing out-of-school physical activity**

Site-Based Interventions: Schools

❁**The Child and Adolescent Trial for Cardiovascular Health** (CATCH)

❁**96 elementary schools in California, Louisiana, Minnesota, and Texas**

❁**CATCH targeted increasing physical activity during physical education classes and outside of school time**

❁**Based on social cognitive theory and organizational change strategies**

Site-Based Interventions: Schools

❁**3rd grade year**

❁**5-week curriculum**

❁**Policy interventions such as the provision of space, equipment and supervision during non-school hours**

❁**Policy and curricula in physical education classes were also introduced**

Site-Based Interventions: Schools

- 4th and 5th grade years

- 12-week curriculum

- Policy components were sustained

- The CATCH project resulted in positive changes in physical activity through the 3 years of the study

- The out-of-school increase in physical activity was still present 3 years later

---

Site-Based Interventions: Worksites

- Worksites have also been targeted environments for physical activity programs

- Expert narrative reviews of literature provided no consensus on the effectiveness of these programs

---

Site-Based Interventions: Worksites

- Dishman and associates (1998) conducted a meta-analysis on 26 studies examining worksite interventions
  - The intervention type was coded as either behavior modification, cognitive behavior modification, health education, health risk appraisal, exercise prescription, or a combination of strategies.
  - Intervention delivery was coded as face-to-face, mediated (indirectly through print or telephone), or a combination of the two, while location was coded as on or off-site.

Site-Based Interventions: Worksites

- The results of the meta-analysis revealed a small positive effect for worksite physical activity interventions

- The size of this effect was not significantly different from zero

- No significant changes to the size of effect based on any of the moderators

- Based upon this meta-analysis it was concluded that worksite physical activity interventions have had little impact

Site-Based Interventions: Health Care Settings

- Simons-Morton and colleagues (1998) provided a review of health care setting physical activity interventions.
  - Physical activity promotion for apparently healthy individuals—Primary Prevention
  - Physical activity promotion for individuals with cardiovascular disease—Secondary Prevention

Site-Based Interventions: Health Care Settings

- 12 primary prevention studies
  - Based on patient counseling
  - No interventions included structured physical activity programs
  - Half were based on an underlying theory
  - 75 % implemented by doctors while nurses or other health professionals administered the remaining interventions.
- The results of these studies were generally positive in the short term
- Effects decreased over time

Site-Based Interventions: Health Care Settings

Simons-Morton et al. (1998) identified 24 studies of physical activity interventions for patients with cardiovascular disease

Only 13 of the 24 studies reported significant changes in physical activity or fitness.

Site-Based Interventions: Health Care Settings

In studies that used an intervention that targeted many risk behaviors (including inactivity), about half were effective in changing physical activity

Based upon the review interventions that included supervised exercise with behavior modification techniques or the provision of home equipment were most often effective (i.e., 75% of the studies)

Community-wide and Policy Interventions

King and collaborators (1995) provided an excellent description of legislative, policy, and environmental approaches to increase physical activity in communities.

➡ Legislation refers to formal legal structures at the local, state, or federal levels of government.

➡ Policy is the formal or informal rules that provide structure to a governing organization.

Community-wide and Policy Interventions

🔔 The Navel Community Project in California

🔔 Three groups: an intervention community, a control community, and a Navy-wide sample

🔔 Cardiovascular fitness was assessed before and after the 1-year intervention period

🔔 The environmental and policy strategies used focused on physical activity and healthy eating

Community-wide and Policy Interventions

🔔 Policy strategies:
- Extending the hours the community recreation center was open
- Communications between superiors and subordinates stressed the expectation that all members of the base should be involved in regular exercise
- Include fruits and vegetables at all snack shops on the Naval base was implemented

Community-wide and Policy Interventions

🔔 Environmental changes:
- New exercise equipment was purchased for the gymnasia
- A women-only fitness center was opened on the base
- 1.5 mile running routes were marked out around the base
- The organization of athletic events and jogging clubs

Community-wide and Policy Interventions

- The intervention had a number of positive benefits for participants who experienced the environmental change condition

- They completed a 1.5-mile run 18 seconds faster following the intervention

- A reduced failure rate during the physical testing (12.4% pre-test down to 5.1% post-intervention)

Community-wide and Policy Interventions

- Did not gain body fat while participants in both control conditions showed significant increases in percent body fat

- Although the number of sedentary individuals (<2000 kcal of activity) increased in all groups, the increase was at a lower rate in the intervention group (about 3%) when compared to the control conditions (about 7%).

Community-wide And Policy Interventions

- Perhaps the most important finding of the study was the extent of the impact for the intervention

- All segments of the population were positively influenced by the intervention strategy thereby providing support for the King et al. (1995) hypothesis that both environmental and policy approaches are effective for increasing physical activity

Mass Media Interventions

- ☼Mass media is often associated with television, radio, and newspapers, but may also included the use of telephones, internet technology, and postal services
- ☼Mass media campaigns
  - ➡ Canada—PARTICIPACTION
  - ➡ United States—Healthstyle
  - ➡ Australia—Life- Be in It
- ☼All have reported increases in population awareness

Recommendations For Community Programs To Promote Physical Activity

- ☼CDC report to summarize recommendations for encouraging physical activity in young people

- ☼The recommendations focused on school and general community programs but most are valuable for, and can be generalized to, any type of community-based intervention

☼END

Chapter 20: A Framework for Evaluating the Public Health Impact of Physical Activity Promotion Interventions

The Psychology of Physical Activity
Albert V. Carron
Heather A. Hausenblas
Paul A. Estabrooks

In theory, there is no difference between theory and practice. In practice there is.
Yogi Berra

The Public Health Impact Of Physical Activity Promotion Interventions

☼ The concern of many health care professionals is the external validity of interventions developed and tested in very controlled environments

☼ Interventions that work in the environment of the randomized clinical control trial are often ineffective in real-world settings

The Public Health Impact Of Physical Activity Promotion Interventions

※ **Why is this so?**
- Resources within real-world settings are different from those in the control trial
- The trained professionals who offered the intervention in the controlled trial were more qualified than those that offer it in a real-world setting

---

The Public Health Impact Of Physical Activity Promotion Interventions

※ The RE-AIM framework was developed by Glasgow and colleagues to determine the public health impact of health promotion intervention and "is concerned with issues related to impact in real-world settings and the translation of research to practice"

The REAIM Framework

※ At the root of the rationale to promote of physical activity is the necessity to improve public health

※ Little is known about the translatability of physical activity programs from research into practice
- Do these things work in the real world?
- Will research be followed by practice?
- How can those people who evaluate physical activity interventions determine if they have had or could have a significant public health impact?

The REAIM Framework

- The RE-AIM framework was developed to evaluate the public health impact of health promotion initiatives

- The RE-AIM framework proposes that the product of an intervention's reach, efficacy, adoption, implementation, and maintenance together provide an indication of an intervention's public health impact.

The REAIM Framework

- Reach--the proportion of the target population that participated in the intervention

- Efficacy--the success in promoting physical activity

- Adoption--the proportion of settings that subsequently uses the intervention

The REAIM Framework

- Adoption--the proportion of settings that subsequently uses the intervention

- Implementation--practitioner's fidelity to the intervention's protocol

- Maintenance--the level of sustained use of the intervention over time

The REAIM Framework

※ Assumes that a public health framework must acknowledge the existence of both individual and organizational levels of impact

※ Reach and efficacy are measured at the level of the individual

※ Reach reflects the number of individuals whereas efficacy reflects the degree to which behavior changes at an individual level

The REAIM Framework

※ Adoption and implementation are organizational levels of impact

※ Adoption is the number of organizations that begin the program and implementation is organizational fidelity to the intervention protocol

※ Maintenance reflects both an individual and organizational level in that the sustained behavior of individuals and organizational use of an intervention can be documented

REACH

※ Proportion of the target population who participate in the initiative

※ Often times the reach of a randomized controlled trail can be determined by the participation rate of those contacted

※ This calculation could overestimate the reach of a given intervention

Reach

- An example: Identifying the reach of a reinforcement intervention to improve attendance at a fitness facility (Courneya, Estabrooks, & Nigg, 1997)

- The study selection criteria included the identification of paying members of the facility who had attended between 4 and 11 times during a random 4-week period

Reach

- 100 randomly selected individuals were then offered a one-month extension to their membership if they attended the facility 12 times over a given 4-week period.
- The reach of a randomized control trial such as this could be computed as 100%.
  - → 100 participants were targeted and subsequently all 100 participants received the intervention.

Reach

- Another calculation of reach would include the entire population of members at the fitness facility (2000 members) who attended 4-11 times over the 4-week selection period

- This new information results in a reach of 5%

- The reach of this study—although high in terms of a research objective—were low in terms of the actual population.

Reach

- In practical terms specific intervention types can be categorized into high, medium or low reach
  - One-on-one in person counseling due to a professional referral=low reach
  - One-on-one counseling delivered as part of regular check-ups =high reach
  - For example, Cheryl Albright and her collaborators (2000) trained 54 physicians to provide sedentary patients with advice on physical activity.
  - Those 54 physicians in turn had contact with 874 sedentary adults.

Efficacy

- During this course we have used findings of many meta-analyses that reported the impact of an intervention through effect sizes
- Effect sizes can be used as a proxy indicator of efficacy
- A higher effect size indicates a more efficacious the intervention
- If an intervention is not efficacious then the issue of reach becomes irrelevant

Adoption

- Adoption is the proportion and representativeness of settings that begin to use the intervention protocol

- It may be useful to refer to the reinforcement study example used previously (Courneya et al., 1997).

- Adoption could be measured by the number of fitness facilities that began to offer a one-month membership extension based on 12 days attended over a given 4-week period

Adoption

- Adoption may be considered the missing link between research and practice
- Research examining physical activity promotion has not documented the success of interventions based upon the adoption of these interventions into mainstream settings
- Effective community based interventions must include mechanisms to ensure adoption of the intervention to various community settings

Adoption

- There are a number of mechanisms to increase adoption
  1) Individuals from all major community groups and institutions should be consulted and informed
  2) Activities should be integrated with existing community activities
  3) Create a systematic plan to constantly identify, recruit, and involve new people and organizations in the project
  4) Summarize and disseminate the results of intervention programs to the participants, community leaders, and important organizations within the community

Implementation

- One concern of physical activity promotion researchers is the extent to which an intervention will be delivered as it was intended
- Implementation is the reflection of the fidelity of practitioners or researchers actions relative to the intended intervention protocol
- The degree of adherence to an intervention protocol has a potential moderating effect on the efficacy of the intervention

Implementation

- The interaction between implementation and efficacy is often described as the effectiveness of the intervention in real-world settings

- Implementation can be measured as treatment fidelity through systematic manipulation checks

---

Implementation

- In smoking cessation it has been shown that a brief hospital-based intervention was more successful when implemented by the research staff when compared to the implementation of the hospital staff

  (Glasgow et al., 1999)

Maintenance

- Maintenance refers to the long-term participation in behavior change and is assessed at both the individual and organizational level

- Typical relapse rates show the need to document the length of adherence to a given positive health behavior

Maintenance

- Many studies include 6-month and 12-month follow-up data points to assess the maintenance of participants' physical activity

- Maintenance can also be examined at the organizational level

- Once a program is started in an organization, its length of existence is seldom reported

Using The REAIM Model As A Practical Evaluation

- The basis of the REAIM framework is to begin with research and evaluate how well that research is translated to the 'real world'

- This is valuable information that can identify gaps in research, such as limited examination of adoption and maintenance at the organizational level

Using The REAIM Model As A Practical Evaluation

- The underlying importance of the RE-AIM framework is the necessity to find interventions that are efficacious and then integrate those interventions across organizational structures (i.e., adoption, implementation) to increase the reach to individuals over an extended period of time (i.e., maintenance)

- How can this information be used to help a physical activity promotion professional?

Using The REAIM Model As A Practical Evaluation

☼ **AN EXAMPLE**

➡ Alison a fictitious director of health promotion for her community

➡ Using the RE-AIM framework Alison could systematically evaluate the programs that are being offered through her community

➡ Alison developed for older adults to become more physically active

➡ The program was implemented at a test facility

Using The REAIM Model As A Practical Evaluation

☼ **Alison could use the REAIM framework to:**

1) Assess the reach of her program for older adults. Within the community she identifies that there are 600 individuals over the age of 65. Currently in her program she has 15 members. Hence, the program's reach is very low (2.5%)

2) Examine the efficacy of her program. She examined the program records and discovers that all of the participants have tripled their weekly minutes of regular physical activity since joining the program—it is efficacious

---

Using The REAIM Model As A Practical Evaluation

☼ **Alison could use the REAIM framework to:**

3) Assess the number of fitness centers that have implemented the intervention. Currently only one program is being offered. Hence, the organizational adoption of the intervention is low

4) View video taped sessions to examine instructor implementation

5) Assess if the the program and the individuals within the program are still ongoing

Using The REAIM Model As A Practical Evaluation

* Alison can now identify major areas in need of attention for her program for older adults

  → she has a program that works very well but she is reaching only a small percentage of the program's target audience--her efforts should be targeting increasing the reach of the program

  → She also determined that there has been no additional organizational adoption of the program. Similarly, efforts could be targeted at marketing the intervention to other communities or organizations

Limitations Of RE-AIM Model

1) It is a descriptive model. The framework provides a very logical way to evaluate programs. It does not provide the processes through which to change the outcomes

2) There is relatively little data to support the claim that each level of the model is equally important

END